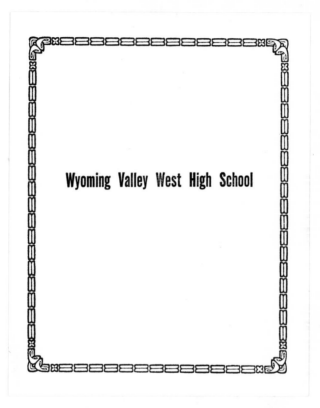

Wyoming Valley West High School

MAYBE YOU DRINK ALCOHOL.

MAYBE YOU DON'T.

EITHER WAY, YOU MAY WANT TO LISTEN TO OTHER TEENAGERS AND FIND OUT:

—How alcohol affects your body

—The most common myths about drinking

—How to handle pressure from your friends

—How to talk to your parents about drinking

—What you can do for a friend—or parent—who drinks too much

—The most dangerous ways to drink

—Why driving while intoxicated is such a problem—and how to avoid it

*Plus* a special section on how to evaluate your own drinking—and where to go for help if you're worried.

# Straight Talk About Drinking

WAYNE COFFEY is a journalist who wrote (under the pseudonym Eric Ryerson) the much acclaimed *When Your Parent Drinks Too Much: A Book for Teenagers*, which was named an Outstanding YA Book of the Year by the American Library Association. He lives in New York City.

# Straight Talk About Drinking
## Teenagers Speak Out About Alcohol

# Wayne Coffey

A PLUME BOOK

**NEW AMERICAN LIBRARY**

A DIVISION OF PENGUIN BOOKS USA INC., NEW YORK
PUBLISHED IN CANADA BY
PENGUIN BOOKS CANADA LIMITED, MARKHAM, ONTARIO

PUBLISHER'S NOTE
The ideas, procedures, and suggestions contained in this book are not intended as a substitute for consulting with your physician. All matters regarding your health require medical supervision.

 PLUME TRADEMARK REG. U.S. PAT. OFF. AND FOREIGN COUNTRIES
REGISTERED TRADEMARK—MARCA REGISTRADA
HECHO EN CHICAGO, U.S.A.

SIGNET, SIGNET CLASSIC, MENTOR, ONYX, PLUME, MERIDIAN and NAL BOOKS are published *in the United States* by New American Library, a division of Penguin Books USA Inc., 1633 Broadway, New York, New York 10019, *in Canada* by Penguin Books Canada Limited, 2801 John Street, Markham, Ontario L3R 1B4

Library of Congress Cataloging-in-Publication Data

Coffey, Wayne R.
    Straight talk about drinking : teenagers speak out about alcohol / Wayne Coffey.
        p.    cm.
    ISBN 0-452-26061-2
    1. Youth—United States—Alcohol use.   2. Youth—United States —Attitudes.   3. Alcoholism—United States—Prevention.   I. Title.
HV5135.C63 1988
362.2'922'088055—dc19                                                87-32446
                                                                            CIP

First Printing, June, 1988

        3    4    5    6    7    8    9

PRINTED IN THE UNITED STATES OF AMERICA

# Contents

# Acknowledgments

More than most, this book was a group effort. The effort came from many different people, and they all deserve heartfelt thanks. My name goes on the cover, but their contributions are what made the project possible.

Special thanks to: the scores of teenagers who offered their time and thoughts, because—very literally—there wouldn't have been a book without them; Dr. James O'Brien, medical director of the alcohol and drug treatment center at the University of Connecticut in Farmington, for sharing his expertise and having the patience to explain it all to a layman; the people at Mark Sheehan High School in Wallingford, Connecticut, for their welcome and their cooperation; Pamela McCarthy-Krombel, a dedicated social worker who was a pleasure to work with and who did yeoman work in arranging many of the interviews; Gordon Greene, for his cooperation and help in recruiting volunteers; and finally, Denise Willi, a very gifted interviewer, whose skillful efforts and unflagging energy—writing, thinking, organizing—were a vital part of the the entire process, and whose moral support was pretty vital, too.

# Straight Talk About Drinking

*Teenagers Speak Out About Alcohol*

# *Introduction*

# THINKING ABOUT DRINKING

The fire was hot. The beer was cold. They were ready.

They were fifteen years old, high school sophomores, and this was going to be their first adventure with alcohol. Everything was set. One of their older siblings had gotten them the beer. They had retreated to their favored hangout, a tree fort tucked in the woods, not far from their neighborhood. They were going to sleep out. They were going to have fun. And they were going to swill their first beers.

There were four of them, and four six-packs on ice. It was a cool, crisp summer evening and the fire was dancing and crackling and soon the beer cans were getting empty. Every time a can went into the discard pile, somebody would say, "Dead soldier," and everybody laughed.

The beer was Schlitz Malt Liquor. The fun was short-lived.

Because not long after the beers were gone, the unpleasantness arrived. There were sick stomachs, pounding heads, and reeling, tipsy bodies. Getting buzzed had spilled over into getting bombed. I know, because one of those pounding heads and sick stomachs belonged to me.

I did dumb things that night. A lot of dumb things. The mistakes, thankfully, were not of the lethal variety; we didn't try to drive in such a state, or go for a ride with anyone else who was. We didn't dodge cars on the highway, and we didn't get into a fight or act like hooligans or vandals. We just stayed around the fire and got annihilated.

Still, it was dumb. I did harm to myself. I made myself sick. I drank and kept drinking, even as the woods began spinning and even though the stuff tasted like motor oil to my inexperienced taste buds. I consumed toxic amounts of a drug—the drug of alcohol—and became incoherent and out of control. On the whole, it was a pretty rotten time. When the hangover arrived the next day, the time got quite a bit worse.

## Plenty of Company

A teenager getting drunk. The experience does not exactly qualify for Ripley's *Believe It or Not*. It's true that teenage drinking is against the law; it's also true that a big percentage of teenagers have done it anyway—and the fifty or so young people interviewed for this book were no different. Perhaps you're no different, either.

I bring up my first drinking experience not because it's unique but because the way I went about it is not unique either. And no matter what your stand on teenage drinking is—whether you think the drinking age is the most ridiculous law in the land or whether you've never had a sip—that's something to be concerned about.

How did I approach that first time? With practically no forethought at all. Pretty much, I just went out in the woods and got wasted. I didn't think about what I was putting into my body. Didn't consider how I might feel afterward. Didn't treat the drug with any respect at all. I just did it.

I said I was dumb that night, and this is why. I took a drug, a whole bunch of it, without giving it a second thought. I did not take the stuff seriously. I should have. Because it *is* serious stuff.

## Hearing from Your Peers

You will get no lectures in this book. You will hear no horror stories concocted with the sole purpose of making you a teetotaler for life, or at least until you reach twenty-one. What you *will* get is a large dose of the thoughts and feelings and attitudes about drinking of people who are probably much like yourself. You will hear from people who are your peers. You will find out what they think about this whole issue, what they think is important, what they're unsure of about alcohol, and what they know.

You'll also get information about alcohol: facts not only about its actual chemical properties and its effect on the human body, but also about myths and misconceptions surrounding it; about dealing with someone—be it family member or friend—whose drinking you're concerned about; about how and why so many people—all of whom are sure they will never have a problem—develop one anyway; and about how and why young people drink. There's more, too.

## A Variety of Voices

There was no elaborate screening process for this interviewing. In fact, there was barely a screening process at all. We did not scour the countryside for teens who would say, "Oh, you should never, ever touch the stuff." We did not look for valedictorians or student leaders or millionaires of tomorrow, and we didn't look for dropouts or lowlifes, either. We only looked for young people who were interested in talking about drinking, and the many issues surrounding it. The looking was easy; almost all of the people you'll soon be hearing from were extremely willing, even eager, interviewees. Their names have been changed, in most instances, only because a good many of them touched on private and personal aspects of their lives.

What we wanted, more than anything, was a cross-section of viewpoints—as representative a sampling as was feasible. We think we've got it. You'll hear from young people whose drinking is a regular part of the social agenda; from people who have not tried it and have no interest in doing so; and from some who drink occasionally. You'll also hear from teenage alcoholics, who share the painful details, with admirable courage and candor, of how their drinking got out of control. We're grateful to all who contributed their time and thoughts to this project, but perhaps most grateful to those for whom the issue is very emotionally loaded. It wasn't easy for them to be questioned about something that has caused them so much pain.

The feeling here is that all those interviewed had a lot of interesting thoughts and insights. We think you'll agree. We also think you'll learn a few things in the pages that follow.

# A Choice to Be Made

The decision to drink is ultimately up to you. So is what and how you drink. Yes, the law has something to say about, and your parents almost certainly do, too. But the reality is that alcohol is everywhere, and it would be folly to pretend that you can't get your hands on it pretty easily if you really want to. So the choice is yours.

The aim of this book is not to influence your decision per se. It's not to rail against alcohol or harangue you about its evils. I happen to drink alcohol. Sometimes I'll have a beer after work. Occasionally I'll have a cocktail when I go out to eat. I've made the decision to drink. And I've made it despite having seen and felt, in full force, the suffering alcohol abuse can cause.

I lived with an alcoholic parent for thirteen years. I felt the hurt and shame and confusion, and watched helplessly as alcohol ravaged the entire family. Nothing has brought more difficulty to my life than alcohol. And yet I drink. I enjoy the taste. It eases me gently into a relaxed mood.

This surprises many people. Others, I know, think it's pretty foolish of me, since it's a proven fact that alcoholism runs in families, that children of alcoholics are four times more likely to develop the disease than the average person.

I don't think it's foolish, however. I've thought a lot about it, and I've learned about it, and I've acquired a huge respect for—and a fear of—what this drug can do. I am careful with it: very careful.

# A Healthy Respect

So what *is* the aim of this book? It is, as the title suggests, to give you good, straight talk on a subject that desperately needs talking about. It's to help you see and understand how your peers feel about the whole issue. But maybe most of all, it's to convey a sense that this substance—this legal, sanctioned, advertised, glamorized substance—deserves your utmost respect. It's to suggest that your decision to drink should be just that—a decision, and a carefully measured one. One that should not be made idly or hastily. It's to get you to do a lot of thinking before you do any drinking.

Even after years of research, we still can't precisely predict who will develop a drinking problem and who won't. Why one so-called social drinker can consume alcohol regularly and never have trouble with it, while another may start the same way and wind up addicted, largely remains a mystery. But there is something else that's not a mystery at all.

And that is that if you go into it with your eyes wide open and your mind aware of how it works and what it can do, if you respect it, you're going to be way ahead of millions of other people, young and old alike. You'll stand a far greater chance of drinking in a way that won't harm you. You'll dramatically decrease the odds of alcohol messing up your life. And you'll dramatically increase your odds of living a better way. A happier, healthier way.

You can get all that just by thinking and weighing, by giving some careful thought to what your peers are saying in the pages that follow. It's a pretty good trade-off, don't you think?

# Chapter 1

# LOOKING AT THE LURE

You don't have to look very hard to find alcohol. If you doubt it, try avoiding it sometime.

How long can you go without hearing or seeing some evidence of drinking? How long without seeing a commercial or a billboard or a magazine advertisement? Without passing a bar or hearing about a drunken-driving accident, or seeing people streaming out of liquor stores, chosen spirits in tow? If you make it an hour, you're either cheating or wearing a blindfold.

If America designated an Official Lubricant, alcohol would be the runaway favorite. Millions of homes are stocked with liquor cabinets. Tens of millions of refrigerators are stocked with beer. Bars are crammed with every intoxicant known to the planet. You can drink on trains, on planes, in health clubs, and at sports events. They even serve alcohol in churches.

Alcohol is also an integral part of social events. Special occasion? Break out the champagne. Got that big raise or straight As on the report card? Hey, let's toast. For Christmas and Thanksgiving, holiday spirits aren't just good feelings: They also come in bottles. People have been known to have a little to drink on New Year's Eve, too.

If teenagers didn't join in with everybody else, this book would not exist and you would probably be reading *Straight Talk About Sex* or *How To Make A Million Dollars Before You're 16*, or some such thing instead. Teenagers are as much a part of this drinking society as anyone else, and the numbers prove it.

One survey showed that 91 percent of teenagers have had alcohol—and more than 50 percent of them have had it by the time they are in ninth grade. Here are some other findings of that survey:

- Eight-five percent of the seniors interviewed had had alcohol in the previous twelve months.
- More than 65 percent had had it in the previous month.
- Nearly a third said that most or all of their friends get drunk once a week.
- Thirty-seven percent said they had five or more drinks in a row at least once in the past two weeks.

There are other numbers that are compiled, too. Tragic ones. Alcohol-related accidents are the leading cause of death among fifteen- to twenty-four-year-olds. Some ten thousand teenagers die every year in alcohol-related accidents. About 4.6 million teenagers have a drinking problem, or have had negative consequences (an accident, a fight, etc.) because of their drinking.

Less serious but still unsavory things can happen as well. Getting caught drinking by your parents, for instance. Getting grounded. Being nabbed for making an illegal purchase. Getting in hot water for showing up at a school dance with a funny smell on your breath. The risks are wide-ranging, and very real.

So what is it about this stuff that makes it so popular? What's the lure here? Why do young people drink in such vast numbers, despite the down side? We asked. We got answers.

## Surefire Fun?

Robert is talking about having fun. He likes having fun. And ever since he's been young, he's seen his family drink to do just that. In his house, drinking was always a quick, convenient way to get happy.

Everybody seemed to enjoy themselves more when they had a few under their belts. Party time meant fun time. And lots to drink.

Robert first drank at a Sweet-Sixteen party. "I was curious. I wanted to see what happened," said Robert. "All my friends drank, so I just wanted to see what it would feel like. So I tried some beers and some screwdrivers. I wasn't drinking that fast. I got buzzed. It was nice, relaxed. I had no hangover the next day."

He enjoyed the warm, happy glow alcohol seemed to bring on. Today, at eighteen, Robert likes going out drinking with his friends about twice a month. Just like those people he grew up with, Robert enjoys the looseness, the euphoria.

"I like to have fun with the guys. A bunch of us will go out in one or two cars. We'll drink beer, wine coolers, schnapps. We just get buzzed, we don't get trashed because we have to go home. We go to the movies, hang out, have fun drinking. I don't know why exactly I think drinking is fun. We fool around more, just see what will happen."

## Heightening the Routine

Without doubt, wanting to have more fun was one of the most popular reasons cited for drinking. For Allison and Weslie, it stems from enhancing more-or-less routine activities.

"It's fun when you're drunk," said Allison. "You do the same things you do every day, except they're just more fun when you're drunk. When you're sober these things don't seem nearly as amusing."

"Yeah, everybody's feeling the same way," added Weslie. "It's fun not being able to walk straight. To get dizzy, doing stupid things. Everyone is screaming and happy, jumping around, everything's more intensified. More funny. Until the next morning. Then it's like, oh my God, pull down the shade."

Rita is friends with Allison and Weslie. She says, "We do have more fun when we're drinking. I admit that. But I don't like it. I wish it weren't true. I wish we could all go somewhere and have fun and not drink, because I'm not sure that it's good to have to drink to have a good time. But I do enjoy it. I do have a better time. You get rowdy. Fun comes more easily."

For Warren, this is the main attraction, too. "It's not that I can't have fun without it. I can go out with my friends, play sports, goof around, and we'll have a good time. But socially, like when you're at a party or something, it sure seems easier to have fun when you've got a few beers inside you. You don't feel as uptight. You're more relaxed, so you see the humor in things more."

Ernie has a different perspective. He thinks there's too

much drinking because there aren't enough other things going on. "I think boredom is a big part of why kids drink," he said. "We get together on the weekends and pool our money and buy some six-packs, and mostly it's not because we're dying to drink, but because we're just bored.

"You drink to have fun, but you do it because you're kind of bored and it's a way to have a good time. You get stupid and you laugh a lot at stupid things. I have to admit, it's more entertaining when you're drinking. But I would by far rather have an action park, with rides and games and stuff, and have it be twenty minutes away and five dollars to get in. It's much better than spending five dollars or six dollars on a six-pack. And it would be a lot more fun."

## The Art of Acting Older

Lauren is fourteen and in the eighth grade. She can hardly wait until next year when she reaches ninth grade; she'll be in high school, and will be able—finally—to hang out with some people other than those her own age. It's one of the reasons she likes to drink.

She drank for the first time in sixth grade. "I was at a friend's house and the parents were gone. A friend of my brother's, he gets the alcohol for me. There were three or four of us, all girls. My brother said, 'Hey, you want some?' and we said yeah, we'll try it. It was Midori (a watermelon liquor). We didn't have much, but it was neat to try, to see if you could get drunk off it or anything. But we didn't; we just got a little buzzed.

"It was daring to do it," said Lauren. "That's how it felt. It was like you were older. You know, more mature, because you're able to drink."

There will be more parties, a busier school agenda, in ninth grade, Lauren figures. "We'll be going out more. We'll meet more guys, be hanging out at these ponds where they have parties all summer long on Friday and Saturday night. There's a lot of drinking there. I just want to go and join in and meet people." Lauren said more girls her age drink than guys, and the reason is simple: The girls are interested in older guys. The older guys invariably drink. So the younger girls go along.

"We all like to be older," said Lauren. "We want to be more sophisticated."

Randi also believes drinking can make you feel more mature. It's what the world tells us, she says.

"I think it was the adults, TV, all of that that made me think that way," she said. "Going to restaurants and seeing older people with these fancy drinks and all the different colors and the limes coming out of the sides. Things like that glamorize drinking a lot, that and magazines, billboards, everything. It kind of makes you think you can't really be adult unless you drink. Like the two go hand in hand."

"When I used to go camping with my older brother and his friends, they would be drinking around the campfire, and I would think it's cool, it's great," added Karl. "I wanted to be just like them. It made me feel grown up."

Martin said that the desire to act older is most strong when you're in junior high. He is eighteen, and says he doesn't care about feeling more adult now. But it was a different story in seventh grade.

"When I was that age, twelve or thirteen, we saw all the big kids we knew who were a year ahead, and we saw them drinking and stuff. You worried that they might not think you were cool kids if you didn't do it also." He wanted to impress the older kids, he said. He wanted to fit in. "When you're that age," said Martin, "it can really be a pressure on you."

## Does Drinking Make the Man?

Just as many girls drink to feel more sophisticated, many guys will do it because they feel it somehow shows they are "real men."

To some people in our society, manhood is measured by one's ability to take a good stiff belt (ice is for wimps) of straight booze, or by being able to hold lots of liquor and remain standing. To some, this qualifies as the height of masculinity.

This notion seems to be fading a little, which is all to the good, because really, what possible connection could there be between someone's masculinity and their ability to pollute their bodies? But it hasn't faded totally, and some of the young men we talked to picked up on it. In particular, they felt being able to drink was a good way to show off in front of the girls.

Take Ernie for example. He wanted to impress a girl he liked, so he raided his parents' liquor cabinet with his brother one day. "I was twelve years old and my parents had gone away. My brother was fifteen or sixteen. We got hammered on beer mainly, but a little bit of everything at my parents' bar. The girl prompted me to do it. I mean, I didn't figure I was going to get all that drunk. Instead, I figured I was a big tough guy. I'd show her. Anything my brother could do, I could do. But he just had a little more practice."

Ernie paid the price. "I hadn't planned on getting sick," he said. "I ended up that night hugging the toilet, praying to the porcelain God." He laughs about it now. That night, it wasn't so amusing.

Karl learned from watching his older brother and his friends pound beers down that drinking is a male ritual. "If they're all drinking, I didn't want to look like a wimp, or like I couldn't handle it or whatever. So I just started drinking harder so I could keep up with them."

Harry is fifteen and said he drank for a while to impress his older buddy, Brandon. Brandon, who is eighteen, had a reputation for being a party animal, a guy who could drink in serious quantity.

"I used to hang out with Brandon a lot, and he used to go to this bowling alley," Harry said. "So I would get drunk for Brandon, just to impress him, mainly. And I was impressed with myself, at the time. I felt, 'Wow, this is great.' I used to do things like climb up a roof and throw stuff down someone's chimney, glasses and stuff, when I was drunk. I'd maybe go through a case of beer without passing out. I would have them one after the other. It would be like a beer every fifteen minutes, then time to have another."

## Unimpressed Observers

Several others related similar stories. Like Ernie, they felt sure their drinking exploits would help them win the favor of various females. It's interesting to note, however, that many of the girls interviewed said they were not impressed in the least; to them, getting drunk and doing outlandish things were not good ways to score points.

"Some guys just want to show off in front of girls. They think it's macho. I don't think it's macho at all, acting stupid," said Joyce. "If they want to impress a girl, they don't have to drink, they can be themselves. If I'm going to like a guy, I'll like him for what he is. I'll like him for his personality, the way he treats me. But if he's going to go and show off, then forget it. I'm not interested."

Clyde isn't interested in selling himself that way, either. "If you really want to meet a girl at a party," he said, "the last thing you want to do is fall flat on your face. Or think that your stool is five feet away from where it is, and fall on the ground accidentally." He thinks alcohol is overrated as a conversational aid, too. "A lot of people think they can't have an interesting conversation unless they're drunk. Of course, they're fooling themselves. When they're drunk they act stupidly. But because everyone else is drunk, they think it's pretty cool."

## The Meet Market: Dating and Drinking

Pat never intended to drink that night. Not much, anyway. It was New Year's Eve, but even so, she wanted to be careful. Maybe have one or two, and that's it.

What Pat didn't count on was to meet this guy. This cute guy. A guy she became interested in very quickly. Pat was thirteen at the time, and plenty nervous.

"I really liked him," she said. "He just handed me a drink and we started talking. Then he handed me another. And then another. He just kept giving me alcohol. It was the first time I had had drinks, except for sipping my dad's beer at home. I had three cans of beer that night, and I don't know what else. The guy just kept giving it to me, and I liked him, so I kept drinking. I just wanted to be with him."

Pat liked that she was feeling more at ease. Slowly her inhibitions began to disappear. Her nerves eased. "Because I was with him, I drank more. I started flirting with him," she said. "I was getting more and more drunk.

I wound up going way overboard. I made a jerk of myself. After that I was embarrassed to see him. The next time we were at the same party I stayed off in the corner.

"I felt pretty good for a while," said Pat with a small laugh. "But then I got drunk. And that was the end of that."

Pat's discovery that alcohol loosens your inhibitions is not unique. It's very natural to feel uneasy and wary about relating to the opposite sex, particularly when you're just starting to date. Alcohol can take the edge off the anxiety; this is what we heard over and over again. Even some older kids felt that way.

Tom and Martin are eighteen. They say they always drink before they try to meet girls at a bar or a disco. "It's easier to pick up girls when you've had something to drink," said Tom. "You have more guts when you have liquor in you. Whenever we go out dancing we'll go out and have a six-pack before we go in to the disco. Then I can walk up to anybody and say, 'Do you want to dance?' And they'll say, 'Sure.' If you're sober and you try to do that you'll go in first, and sit down. Have some drinks, but sit there and watch the girls because you have no guts. But with a few beers in you, you're bold."

Also, rejection seems much easier to take, Martin said. "If they say 'Get lost, get out of here we don't want to dance with you,' it doesn't bother you as much," he said. "It's more like, 'Oh well, then, it's your loss.' If I was sober and I got turned away I would feel like crawling under a chair and leaving. I would feel like crap."

For Warren, alcohol is sort of like adding oil to a machine. "It just makes me looser and frees things up," he said. "I get very self-conscious when I'm talking to a girl at a party. I get thinking too much and worry about whether I'm going to say something dumb or whether she'll like me. And it doesn't feel so much that way after I've had a little to drink.

"But I don't know if it's worth it. Because it isn't that far from this being-loose state, and being drunk and acting like a jerk. Then nobody's going to want to be with you."

While drinking may make you feel more confident with someone you're attracted to, there's also the possibility that you might become too comfortable with the opposite sex and go overboard, warned Joyce. You might fool around, even if you don't want to. You might end up going much further than you want to.

Joyce knows what she can be like when she loses control of her senses. She doesn't always trust herself, so she's very cautious. "When I drink I get crazy. I'm a very hyper person to begin with. When I drink I loosen up even more. If a guy came on to me, I wouldn't know if I'd be able to stop them if I were buzzed. I don't even want to find out what would happen. I might get into serious trouble if I wasn't thinking clearly." Joyce's wariness is well-placed; a high percentage of teenage pregnancies *do* occur when one or both parties have had alcohol.

## The Great Escape?

Life has gotten pretty tough for Stan. His parents recently divorced. Living with his father, who is an active alcoholic, has been almost unbearable at times. To make matters worse, Stan's dad lost his job because of his drinking. Just being home, thinking about all the stuff that's going on, it's enough to get Stan twisted up in knots. He has never felt this tense, this depressed, in his whole life.

When the pressure gets really bad, Stan has found an escape. He drinks.

"I'd say I drink about once a month, if I have had a tough time in school or a rough day at home," he said. "I'll have a few, one or two beers at home by myself to ease the tension of things. It relaxes me."

Stan is fourteen. He had his first drink when he was in fifth grade. "I snuck a beer. I just opened up the refrigerator and took one to see what it was like. I didn't really like the taste of it. I thought beer was bitter and sour." Then, this year he learned what it was like to get drunk.

A group he belongs to had a convention in a hotel. They spent the night partying, five teenagers and an adult supervisor who was not doing much supervising.

"We had four cases of beer to drink, and left just half a case when the party was over," said Stan. "I didn't have to get home until three-thirty the next afternoon, so I just kept going. I think I drank twelve beers in all. I know I couldn't stand up, but I didn't black out. All I know is that I just felt good, I didn't have any worries. I was relaxed for a change."

The next day brought an awful hangover, but it was worth it, Stan said. He doesn't think he'll get that drunk again soon. But he liked not being weighted down with worries about the stuff going on at home. "I had a good time," he said.

Stan's friend Karl also gets drunk to get away from the hassles at home. Karl says he does it as often as he can. "When I'm drunk, I just forget about how things are going or whatever. It's seems to relax me, makes me more at ease."

For Karl there's a direct correlation between how upset he is about things and how often he wants to drink.

"I have more problems, things I'm worried about right now. I just feel like getting drunk more. To relax or something, just get out of it for a little while. That's how I look at it."

Lisa also felt upset about things going on at home. "That's why I drank. The first time was just for fun, but after that, I'd see my father come home drunk every night, and I'd be sick of it. My parents would get in a big fight. Usually it was over something I did or didn't do. Why should I listen to this? That was my attitude. Drinking was an escape."

Lisa also said, "I was aware of wanting to get back at them." The more she talked, the clearer became the deep anger she feels toward her parents—because she feels they don't care, that they never give her support or credit for anything. "Sometimes I'd say to myself, well, I'll come home drunk, too, and see how they like it."

## Escaping into Trouble

There is something very dangerous about drinking as an escape—and we heard about the dangers from a number of those who drank for that reason. They talked about slowly, subtly sensing they were becoming more dependent on alcohol. They talked about how, the more they relied on drinking as a way of handling things, the less able they were to deal with things when they were sober. It's kind of like being out of shape physically: If you haven't kept yourself fit, and then go out and try to run two miles, it's going to be much tougher than if you had been in condition all along. Our ability to cope with problems also can get out of condition.

They also talked about how the escape, no matter how appealing it seemed, provided extremely short-term relief for their troubles. Here's Weslie: "You get drunk because you want to forget about everything. You want to be deranged. I don't want to see life the way I do when I'm sober. I want a change, a change from the boring, from the pressures on your shoulders, your parents, school, everything. But what I found out was that it would always backfire. I'd feel better for a little while, but then you come down, and it's much worse than it was before."

Weslie learned the lesson the hard way. She drank one night when she was upset about things. She got pretty drunk—and really depressed. "It was scary," she said. "I didn't care about anything. I just couldn't deal with it." She spoke of feeling very alone, very overwhelmed. Of finding out what we looked at earlier—that alcohol is a depressant, a very potent one, indeed.

"You're depressed when you're drunk. The happiness wears off, and then it's like being in a vacuum. Like nobody is there. Nobody cares. Nothing matters. You could die tomorrow and nobody cares. It's the worst feeling. You have all these problems and you have no idea what to do about them. Everything runs through your head. You just want to scream.

"So that's it," said Weslie. "After that, never again. I'm feeling depressed now, and I won't drink. I'm not going to go through that again."

Arlene has made a similar realization. "If I didn't want to face my problems, I used to drink. Kids would say, 'Here take it. This will make you happy.' I'd be at a party and I'd drink and get really drunk. And it's stupid, actually. I should never do that, because when I got over the hangover my problems were still there."

Karl, too, is starting to acknowledge the dangers of the alcohol escape. "It just changes your attitude about things, can mess you up," he said. "In some ways it helps relieve the tension, but that doesn't last. That's why people overdo it. That's how people become alcoholics."

For Pat, it's pretty clear: You drink to escape problems, and then the drink is gone and the problems are still there. "Most people you see drink, they want to drown themselves and forget their problems," she said. "But I just think if I go out and drink every time I have a problem, it'll be there the next day, and then I'll want to get drunk again. You get nowhere."

## The Pressure Points

The invitation arrived, and Shirley was psyched. It was going to be her first chance to check out a high school party. She was thirteen, and as the day drew closer, she was more and more excited about it.

The party was at a friend's house, and it promised to be a wild night. Her girlfriend's older brother was inviting all his high school junior and senior friends. And his parents were going to be away all weekend.

When she arrived, Shirley realized she was one of the youngest people there. The music was loud, and the older kids were all clutching beers and plastic cups of high-powered punch and were well on their way to getting loaded. Suddenly Shirley got nervous. She realized she had never been a part of something like this before.

"We got there a little late," said Shirley, "and as soon as we did, someone offered us some beer. All my girlfriends said 'Yeah, yeah, I'll take some.' So I figured I might as well take some also."

At first, Shirley was reluctant to drink. She was afraid, terrified actually, of what would happen if her parents smelled booze on her breath. Or worse, caught her being drunk.

Shirley said she really didn't want to drink that night.

But she decided to anyway—despite her own feelings, despite her worries about her parents. She did it because she wanted to fit in, be part of the crowd.

"It was pressure really that made me decide to drink," she said. "Everyone else was doing it, so it was like, why not? Plus you worry about what people are thinking, like, 'She's got to go home to her mom,' or something like, 'It figures, she wouldn't be drinking.' So I began drinking beer, and some wine and stuff. I felt kind of weird, and funny and giggly and maybe disorderly a little. I had never gotten drunk before."

Wanting to join the crowd can be a powerful influence; it was far and away the most common—and most compelling—reason we heard for drinking. You don't want to feel out of the social flow. You don't want people to think you're some kind of infant. You want to have fun like everybody else. You just don't want to be different, because sometimes it's really hard to be different. So you drink—whether you really, truly want to or not.

Sometimes the pressure can be subtle, and self-imposed. As Lisa explained, "I think it's the crowd that usually gets me drinking. The first time I drank I was at a Saint Patrick's Day celebration at the firehouse with my parents. All the guys were eighteen, and I was the youngest kid there. There were two kegs, and other stuff like vodka and whiskey. People were doing shots. My father was beyond help, and my mother was on her way there. I was sitting in the back of a fire truck and I just started drinking with them. It was really weird. I was in sixth or seventh grade and everybody was five or six years older. And I just started drinking with everybody. I looked around and everybody was trashed. I said, this is really exciting. Give me a drink, maybe I can be happy too."

Nobody overtly pressured Lisa. But she was at the party and she wanted to fit in. So she went for it.

## High-Pressure Tactics

Sometimes the pressure is much more blatant, as in Martin's case. "At the end of eighth grade I remember going up behind a neighborhood church," he said. "Some kids were drinking, but I didn't really care to drink. It was the last day of school. They just kept taunting me, 'Come on. You're going to be a freshman next year. Come on, Martin.' "

He resisted at first. But they kept at it. Kept badgering him to join in, and finally Martin relented. "I drank maybe four or five beers, a couple of shots of Southern Comfort, and some vodka that they were drinking. And I got mighty sick, the first time that had ever happened. I didn't drink because I liked the alcohol. I drank because everybody else was doing it, because they pressured me. I was thinking all the time, 'I don't want to drink. I want to go home now.' My parents never smelled it. I didn't get caught, thank God."

The pressure weighs on everybody at one time or another, but perhaps it's most intense when you're in the early teens, in junior high; when the feeling of wanting to belong, to be accepted, to be cool, is very strong. Alcohol, for many, is the best and fastest way to meet it.

"I think it's toughest when you're younger," said Pat. "Even before seventh or eighth grade, you feel the pressure. You're just starting out and you don't know how to handle yourself." She paused and then continued. "Maybe you want to impress your friends and show them you can drink at an early age. And when you get older, and you're hanging around these cool kids and stuff, you can say, 'Well, I've been drinking since I was eleven years old.' Some people will go, 'Wow. Really, eleven?' "

Laurie agreed. "When you get older the pressure gets less. By freshman year, you know more what to do, what you want. I haven't had any problems or anything."

Ellen is seventeen now but remembers eighth grade vividly. "I was at this party, and some kids were smuggling in stuff. Soon almost everybody was drinking. I didn't want to drink, and I would make up excuses about why. I couldn't just say I didn't want it, because they kept pushing and pushing. You know, 'Go ahead, try it, it isn't going to hurt you. Look at us. We're drinking and we're having a lot of fun.' "

Another time, a close friend of Ellen had a party. The friend went on a full-scale effort to get Ellen to drink. "She said, 'You'll have such a good time. Have some Schnapps or Peachtree or whatever you want, you'll feel so much better. Don't worry about it. We'll drive you home. We'll take care of you. We'll have a great time.' "

## Their Persistence, Your Resistance

Ellen's experience is very common; her response, however, was very rare: She didn't buckle under. She did not care to drink and she stood by her conviction. "I lost a few friends because of it," she said. "But that's okay. It worked out for the best. And as I got older, it got much easier to resist that kind of pressure."

Whether you decide to drink or not is an extremely important—and personal—decision. It's a decision to be made by you, nobody else. Many teenagers choose to drink of their own accord, for their own particular reason. Some choose not to.

What if you're among those who prefer not to drink

right now? The reason doesn't matter. Maybe you don't like the taste. Maybe you have a parent or older brother or sister who has run into trouble with drinking, or you've seen how other kids act after drinking and you don't care for it. Or maybe you just don't think it's right for you. Period. Whatever the reason, it is absolutely your right—and all right—to not drink. So what do you do when some of this pressure we've been talking about comes your way? What happens when your friends are egging you on, telling you not to be a party pooper, guaranteeing you'll enjoy it and be fine? How do you wait until you're ready?

Bob is fourteen and in the eighth grade. He's had a few sips of wine and beer but doesn't really like the taste. He also doesn't like what alcohol can do to people who abuse it, he said. His alcoholic stepfather, who has since left home, often had violent mood swings.

"He used to come up to me in the middle of supper, after he had been drinking, then he'd yell at my mom and scream at me, 'Why did you do this and why did you do that?' " Bob said. "My mom told me, 'I don't want you to ever be like him.' So I don't drink at all."

Bob has friends who drink quite a bit. They used to pressure him a lot, he says. "Because I wouldn't drink or smoke, they would call me 'wimp' or 'baby.' But I just walked away," Bob said. "It didn't matter to me. It's my own life, and I'll take care of it my way. Most of the stuff they said wasn't true anyway. They were the ones being stupid, not me."

Sticking to what you think is best for you, recognizing that your opinion counts more than anyone else's, is one way to tackle pressure from friends. It made Bob feel good about himself. It was hard, sure. But he was glad he was able to walk away.

"I just came to myself one day and said, 'Why do I

have to be like everyone else? I'm my own individual.' I can go out on my own."

Bob did just that. He stopped hanging around with his old friends. He found some new ones, a few very loyal guys with whom he shares a similar viewpoint. "I only have three or four friends, but they are real friends. Everyone else cheats on you. They aren't loyal friends. They made fun of me. What kind of a friend is that?"

His new friends never try to impose their values or attitudes on him, he says. "My best friend, Larry, he looks like a girl because he has long hair, but he's not. We usually do a lot of things like go to the arcade, or shopping or something. We like mostly the same things. My friends, they wouldn't even try to tell me to drink something. They're not that kind of people. They don't agree with drinking."

Though it hurt to be excluded by some of his former friends, Bob feels good that he was strong enough to do what he felt was right. "Everyone in my grade who drinks does it because they think it's cool," he said. "They want to be like everyone else. Be part of a group, wear the same clothes, have the same hairstyles. Drink, smoke. Well, I don't like all those things. That's why I'm different. You don't see many people wearing their hair this way, or these kind of shirts. Everyone always comes up to me and says, 'Oh, what a tacky shirt.' " Bob pointed to his loud print shirt and punk-style haircut. "But I like it."

## Alternative Activities

Evan is fifteen and doesn't drink anymore. He loved the taste of alcohol, but couldn't always stop drinking when he wanted to, and that made him afraid. His drinking was interfering with his home life and at school. When he decided he wanted to stop, his first step was to stop going to the usual drinking hangout—the bowling alley.

The environment and the pressure to drink were just too powerful a tug on him. "I figured that I know if I go down there I'm going to get drunk. So I didn't," Evan said.

Instead, he started doing other things. He formed a band—all of whose members have taken a vow not to drink or take drugs. The band members used to drink a lot; all wanted to stop.

Evan makes no mistake about the difficulty of avoiding the pressure to drink. "It's really hard," he said. "Everywhere you look there's somebody with alcohol in their hands, asking you if you want some. And you're saying, 'No, it's okay,' and half the time you're sweating it out because you really want some." For Evan, one of the keys to fighting off the pressure is to hang around with the right people. "Half the time I think kids want to fit in with a certain crowd, so they just go along with them. They want to feel cool. That's more important to them than anything." Evan paused. And he said, "Drinking isn't going to make you cool. That has nothing to do with it."

Ernie doesn't think so either. Which is why he had to confront a friend of his at a party. This guy is older, twenty-three, and he's always getting drunk, Ernie said. "There's one in every crowd—you know, the guy who gets hammered and is always trying to force it on everyone else." The guy was very insistent this one night, practically sticking a beer in Ernie's face, all the while saying to him, "What are you, a Mama's boy?"

Ernie did not give in. He told the guy to back off. "If you don't want it, you just say no," Ernie said. "No one can force you to drink. I've never met a kid at a party who's going to knock you over and pour it down your throat. And usually the people who are doing the forcing are the people you hear apologies from the next day. They say, 'Oh, I'm sorry, I didn't mean to get like that.' So who's going to look like a jerk the next day? You, for not drinking? Or the guy who's all drunk and forcing it on you?

"That makes you see why you should stick to your guns," Ernie went on. "That's how I look at it. I look at the kid and I think, 'I'm going to chug this beer so I can be like you? No thanks.' " Being able to do this gives Ernie a lot of satisfaction. "You know you're doing what you think is right. Inside, it feels good."

## Friends: The Fake Kind, the Real Kind

Maggie also has worked at not letting others sway her. She drinks mostly on special occasions, and wants it to stay that way. She says she doesn't worry about being an outcast, or what so-called friends think of her decision.

"These people who feel you have to drink—and who pressure you to drink—are really fake friends," said Maggie. "If they can't respect your opinion, then they aren't your friends."

Nobody we talked to said fighting off this pressure was easy. On the contrary, they said it was very hard. What makes it especially hard is that often those doing the pressuring are your friends, and usually they feel they have your best interest at heart. They may truly think you will feel better if you have a nip or two. They may think it would do you good to mellow out and loosen up, and that alcohol is the way to do it. They may even think it shows their loyalty as a friend if they help you get drunk and then watch over you.

This is one case where good intentions count for very little, however. Even if it's your best friend doing the leaning, you're best off paying mind only to yourself, and your own needs. You'll wind up respecting yourself a lot more—this is the message we heard over and over again. And if a friend is put off or going to get bent out of shape about that, well, that is his or her problem.

Resisting peer pressure isn't easy. But every person we interviewed said it was well worth it. Martin put it well: "There's no reason to do it if you don't want to. If you *want* to try it, fine. But if you don't, there's no reason. Nobody should hassle you if you just look them right in the eye and say, 'I really don't feel like it.' If they can't see that, they're really not worth having as friends. Who wants friends who can't understand your feelings?"

# Chapter 2

# ALCOHOL:
# What It Is, What It Does

Imagine stopping by a car dealership. You look around, and you see one gleaming hunk of transportation after another. You see all kinds of them, all over the place. You see different shapes and sizes, different makes and colors. You see slow cars and fast cars, dull cars and jazzy, frilly cars. The variety is practically endless.

Now think of walking into a liquor store. You will not see any cars (unless a drunk plowed into the store window), but you will see the same bewildering array of varieties. You will see liquor packaged in all manner of shapes and sizes; liquor made in the Soviet Union, wine made in France or Italy or Chile, and maybe beer made in a brewery in your own state.

Just as there is a car to suit everyone's style, there is booze for everyone's palate. You can get stuff that's sweet and syrupy and peach-flavored, or you can get something that's thin and colorless and so powerful it will knock off your socks and possibly your shoes. You can also get any number of beverages in between.

There are hundreds of kinds and brands of alcoholic beverages. Other than being wet, they all have one main thing in common: At bottom, they're all a chemical substance called ethyl alcohol, or ethanol. Just as beneath all the automotive jazz—the racing stripes and cassette decks and sunroofs—a car is basically an engine and wheels, liquor is basically juiced-up, jazzed-up ethyl alcohol.

We've looked at the reasons why people drink. Now let's look at what it is they are drinking, at what ethyl alcohol is, what it does (and can do), and how it affects the human body.

## The Basics

Alcohol, first and foremost, is a drug. It is a chemical compound; ethyl alcohol's scientific makeup is $C_2H_5OH$ (two carbon molecules, five hydrogen molecules, and a hydroxyl group), and it is made from such substances as grains or fruit or potatoes. Beer is made by breaking down, or fermenting, various grains. Wine is made by fermenting fruit, usually grapes. And so-called hard liquor—vodka, whiskey, rum, gin, etc.—is made by heating a fermented substance, separating the alcohol from the water, and then collecting the alcohol in recondensed form. The process is called distillation.

Alcohol has been around for thousands of years. Explicit references to it are found as far back as 4000 B.C., when some folks in Mesopotamia filled clay tablets with their favorite wine recipes. There are also more than 150 alcohol references in the Bible, including the book of

Proverbs, where it is written, "Wine is a mocker, strong drink is raging; and whosoever is deceived thereby is not wise." In the Chinese *Canon of History*, dating to roughly 650 B.C., it says that "men will not do without beer," so trying "to prohibit it and secure total abstinence from it is beyond the power even of the sages." In ancient Babylonia, around 1700 B.C., the Code of Hammurabi laid down restrictions about when and where alcohol could be consumed.

Throughout history, there are testimonials to what alcohol can do for you. There are also references aplenty to what it can do *to* you. Drinking and drinking problems apparently were an item right from the start.

## The Body's Slowdown

Alcohol is a depressant. It slows down the body's central nervous system, which includes the brain, the spinal cord, and the nerves connected to them. The nervous system is the hub of the human body, and liquor reduces all functions related to it. This means that alcohol hinders our judgment, physical sensations, emotional functioning, motor skills, speech, learning ability, and memory. Precisely how it does all this is more the stuff of a biology text than this book; suffice it to say that when alcohol seeps into the central nervous system, it disrupts our nerve cells and impairs the flow of the electrical impulses that make the whole system work. Alcohol is potent stuff. Very potent.

## The False Buzz

Many of those interviewed were surprised to learn that alcohol is a depressant. "I get all hyper when I drink," said Gina, who is thirteen. "I feel like I've got more energy than normal."

It's a common misconception that liquor stimulates you, because you often feel looser, funnier, have more powerful feelings when you've had a little to drink. Even the popular slang words for getting drunk—buzzed, juiced, bombed, high, hammered, loaded—give a sense of a revved-up, stimulated effect.

But the words fool you, says Dr. James O'Brien, medical director of the alcohol and drug treatment center at the University of Connecticut in Farmington, with whom we consulted in preparing this chapter.

"A lot of people think it's a stimulant," Dr. O'Brien said. "And the reason is that when we drink, alcohol actually depresses the part of the brain, the so-called higher center, that governs our inhibitions." Thus we become more uninhibited, and tend to do things we might not do ordinarily. We feel an initial surge of a carefree kind of energy.

"People often interpret this as stimulation," Dr. O'Brien said, "but it's really the depression of the brain." As the drinking continues, the slowdown becomes more pronounced. Before long, the ability to speak, think, and respond is markedly lessened. All the functions of the central nervous system are dulled.

"Alcohol is a total anesthetic," said Dr. O'Brien. "If I could give it to you by vein, I could take out your gall bladder, using just alcohol as an anesthetic." Alcohol is that good at numbing pain.

In fact, the slowdown alcohol causes in the body can be so extreme that if you have enough, your respiratory system will just stop. Breathing gets slower and slower the more you drink. And finally, it can quit altogether. At which point you die.

You have to drink quite a bit to reach this stage. "But

it takes a lot less than people think," said Dr. O'Brien. "There are so many people out there who have no intention of doing any harm to themselves, but who have no idea how fast it can hit them."

How fast is fast? If your blood alcohol level reaches .32 percent, you are endangering your life, says Dr. O'Brien. And what does it take to reach .32 percent? We'll look at what blood alcohol level is (and how to figure it) shortly, but if you weigh, say, 150 pounds and you have two six-packs of beer—twelve twelve-ounce bottles—your level would be roughly .29. You would be very drunk—and not very far from trouble. Seven stiff drinks (with two ounces of alcohol apiece) would put you in the same incoherent neighborhood.

## The Proof Is on the Label

The stronger the liquor, the more numbing it does. The strength of alcohol is expressed in proof, which you will see on the label of distilled liquor. Proof measures the amount of absolute alcohol in a given beverage. The term "proof" is centuries old and stems from people wanting just that—proof—that the booze they were drinking had the proper percentage of alcohol. Various tests were devised to make the determination; five hundred years ago, for instance, people would float oil on top of liquor, and if the oil sank that was proof the alcohol content was adequate. Another test was to light an alcohol-soaked cloth. If it burned easily and quickly, that, too, was proof.

The percentage of alcohol in a drink is exactly half of its proof. Thus, if you have 80 proof vodka, you're drinking a substance that is 40 percent alcohol. If you have beer that is 8 proof, it is 4 percent alcohol. Wine that is 22 proof would contain 11 percent alcohol.

## Alcohol at Work

Some people think of alcohol as food in liquid form. It is not. Its food value is zero. It has no protein, minerals, or vitamins. It has nothing but calories, and quite a few of them: about 150 in a twelve-ounce beer, 100 in a five-ounce glass of wine, 100 in a one-ounce portion of hard liquor.

Because alcohol is not food, it does not need to be digested. You ingest it and it goes through the stomach and the intestinal wall and spews into the bloodstream, which carries it to the brain and all parts of your body. This is why we feel the effects of alcohol fairly quickly. It makes no detours.

The only organ in the body that can metabolize, or break down, alcohol is the liver. A very small percentage of alcohol is gotten rid of through perspiration, saliva, and breath. The rest—95 percent of it—is handled by the liver, which breaks it down into carbon dioxide and water.

The breakdown happens slowly. "You process alcohol at a very standard rate," said Dr. O'Brien. "A young drinker can burn off at best two-thirds of an ounce of hundred proof alcohol per hour." Or two-thirds of a can of beer, or of a five-ounce glass of wine. If you drink faster than that—even if you have, say, two beers per hour (not considered a rapid rate by most people)—your blood alcohol level will continue to rise. And you will get drunk, because your alcohol intake is outstripping the pace of your liver in breaking it down.

This deliberate breakdown means that the amount of

alcohol inside you is greater than you think. It also means that the alcohol continues to get absorbed in your bloodstream even after you've stopped drinking. The result is that your blood alcohol level keeps going up for a while. And you get much drunker than you figured you would.

We tend not to think of four drinks over two hours as a vast amount of drinking. Yet there's an excellent chance you will be legally intoxicated with this much in you (that is, your blood alcohol level will be .10 percent or higher), and it's 100 percent certain your ability to drive will be impaired, even if you are under the .10 mark. Tests have shown that, at .07 percent, most teenagers will have some trouble talking, have slurred speech, and begin showing signs of real intoxication. They also have shown that, no matter how sober we may feel, our abilities to judge and react are markedly decreased with just .05 percent alcohol in the blood. In fact, the odds of having an accident are double what they would be normally with this .05 percent alcohol level inside us.

That .05, for a 150-pound person, amounts to little more than two twelve-ounce beers. Alcohol hits faster—and harder—than we know. And it hits teenagers faster still. "We don't really know precisely why," said Dr. O'Brien, "but teenagers seem to get intoxicated at a lower blood alcohol level."

## Facts and Figuring

Knowing about the blood alcohol level is important. Not only does it help us understand how much more we're affected than we may think, it also is a good safeguard against driving or swimming, or doing anything else we're not in shape to do. If you know that at .20

blood alcohol level you would be extremely out of it (which you or I or anybody else definitely would be), and know what it takes to get there, you can ease off before serious trouble arrives.

Blood alcohol concentration is simply a measurement of the amount of alcohol in a given quantity of blood. As we've seen, a legal state of intoxication is usually .10 percent alcohol in the blood. (This is the law in most states; in a few, however, it's .08, and there has been talk that .10 is really too high a cutoff and that other states are considering dropping to .08 as well.) If you know your weight and how much you've had to drink (or plan to drink), you can figure out your blood alcohol level quite easily. The formula is:

$$150/\text{your weight} \times \text{alcohol percentage}/50 \times \text{no. of fluid ounces} \times .025$$

Let's say you weigh 150 pounds. And that you have five cans of beer that is 4 percent alcohol. Your five cans amount to sixty ounces of drink. Using the formula, we would calculate this way:

$$150/150 \times 4/50 \times 60 \times .025$$

And you would get a blood alcohol level of .12 percent. Which would mean you should get nowhere near the wheel of an automobile.

As another example, let's say you had three five-ounce glasses of wine. The wine was 11 percent alcohol. Back to the formula:

$$150/150 \times 11/50 \times 15 \times .025$$

And you would get .0825 as your blood alcohol level. You wouldn't be legally drunk. But it still would be a very poor idea to get near the wheel.

If math isn't your bag, take it easy. We've got a chart that will let you determine your approximate blood alcohol level without getting into the number-crunching.

Another fact worth noting is that, because of the slow breakdown we discussed, blood alcohol level decreases only .015 per hour. Thus, if a friend gets really tanked and you figure he has a .15 blood alcohol level, even after three hours of sobering up, he would still be at .105—over the legal drunk limit. Which means you keep him far away from the wheel, too.

## Food for Thought

Warren was talking about a recent bout of drinking. He said, "I had pretty much to drink, but I didn't get drunk because I made sure I had a nice, big meal beforehand." Donna related the opposite experience. She went to a party, had practically nothing in her stomach, and had several drinks in succession. "I got really drunk," she said, "and I would've barely been buzzed if I had made sure I'd eaten something."

I remember thinking the same way about food. I assumed it made all the difference, because the older kids would always make a big deal about having something in your stomach before drinking. One kid I knew even talked about *what* you ate being the key; he insisted buttermilk, taken before drinking, would coat your stomach and thus alcohol wouldn't affect you as much.

---

For the most accurate reading, once you have the blood alcohol reading for your sex, weight, and number of drinks, subtract .015 for every hour you have been drinking. Thus, if you are a 125-pound female who has had four drinks in two hours (a drink equaling one twelve-ounce can of beer, a five-ounce glass of wine, or a half ounce of distilled alcohol (vodka, gin, whiskey, etc.), you would subtract .030 (.015 × 2) from .162. You would get .132. And you would be drunk.

---

## ESTIMATED BLOOD ALCOHOL LEVELS

### Males

| Ideal Body Weight (lbs.) | Number of Drinks | | | | | | | | | |
|---|---|---|---|---|---|---|---|---|---|---|
| | 1 | 2 | 3 | 4 | 5 | 6 | 7 | 8 | 9 | 10 |
| 100 | .043 | .087 | .130 | .174 | .217 | .261 | .304 | .348 | .391 | .435 |
| 125 | .034 | .069 | .103 | .139 | .173 | .209 | .242 | .278 | .312 | .346 |
| 150 | .029 | .058 | .087 | .116 | .145 | .174 | .203 | .232 | .261 | .290 |
| 175 | .025 | .050 | .075 | .100 | .125 | .150 | .175 | .200 | .225 | .250 |
| 200 | .022 | .043 | .065 | .087 | .108 | .130 | .152 | .174 | .195 | .217 |
| 225 | .019 | .039 | .058 | .078 | .097 | .117 | .136 | .156 | .175 | .195 |
| 250 | .017 | .035 | .052 | .070 | .087 | .105 | .122 | .139 | .156 | .173 |

### Females

| Ideal Body Weight (lbs.) | Number of Drinks | | | | | | | | | |
|---|---|---|---|---|---|---|---|---|---|---|
| | 1 | 2 | 3 | 4 | 5 | 6 | 7 | 8 | 9 | 10 |
| 100 | .050 | .101 | .152 | .203 | .253 | .304 | .355 | .406 | .456 | .507 |
| 125 | .040 | .080 | .120 | .162 | .202 | .244 | .282 | .324 | .364 | .404 |
| 150 | .034 | .068 | .101 | .135 | .169 | .203 | .237 | .271 | .304 | .338 |
| 175 | .029 | .058 | .087 | .117 | .146 | .175 | .204 | .233 | .262 | .292 |
| 200 | .026 | .050 | .076 | .101 | .126 | .152 | .177 | .203 | .227 | .253 |
| 225 | .022 | .045 | .068 | .091 | .113 | .136 | .159 | .182 | .204 | .227 |
| 250 | .020 | .041 | .061 | .082 | .101 | .122 | .142 | .162 | .182 | .202 |

—Robert O'Brien and Morris Chafetz, M.D.,
The Encyclopedia of Alcoholism (Facts on File, Inc.)

Many of the interviewees had the same belief about food. Many looked at it as a surefire safeguard against drunkenness. But Dr. O'Brien says it isn't. It isn't that at all. The physiological reality is simply that although food does slow the rate at which alcohol hits the bloodstream, it does nothing more than slow it. Food doesn't block alcohol, or soak it up. It doesn't counteract its effects. It only gives the booze something else to pass through before moving along through your body.

Nor can food do anything special for you after you've been drinking. Said Dr. O'Brien, "Many people think that it helps if you eat bread or something after drinking. They think the alcohol in their stomachs is like alcohol sitting in a dish, and that bread will absorb it all and sober them up. That really isn't true."

Does this mean it doesn't matter if you drink on an empty stomach? Not at all. It's not a good idea to drink that way, because the alcohol will race into your system and hit you much more quickly. You will get drunker faster, and if you keep drinking, you can reach a dangerously high blood alcohol level so much the sooner. The point is simply that as Dr. O'Brien notes, "Food will not protect you. You will absorb all the alcohol you take in. The process will just happen more slowly."

## Slaying Some Other Myths

If you've done any drinking, or been around people who have, you've undoubtedly heard about various schemes for getting sober. You've heard about drinking hot coffee, taking a cold shower, going for a walk, or maybe drinking a lot of water.

These are but a few of the most popular drying-out ploys after having a little (or a lot) too much to drink.

None of them work. They can make you more awake. They can not make you more sober.

Drinking coffee may be the most popular of all. To a lot of people, it's almost a magical sobering agent; drink all night, but have a couple cups of coffee before you leave and you'll be fine. "If you give someone coffee after they're drunk," said Dr. O'Brien, "all you will have is an alert drunk. Coffee is a stimulant, but the person is still intoxicated."

And a cold shower? "A cold shower gives you a clean drunk," said Dr. O'Brien. The fact is, nothing you do to get sober faster will do any good, because the rate at which you get sober is the rate at which your liver breaks down the alcohol. And that cannot be speeded up. Not by the coldest shower, the strongest coffee ever brewed, or anything else. You want to get sober, you only need one thing: time. A lot of it. The liver does nice work. It just does it at its own pace.

## Holding Your Liquor

You may know a large, well-muscled person who seems to be able to consume significantly more alcohol than everyone else. This isn't your imagination.

The bigger and stronger you are, the more alcohol you can drink before getting drunk. The reason is simple: Big, strong people have more water in their bodies. They have more water not just because of their size, but because of their muscle mass. Muscles retain a greater percentage of water than fat does. This allows powerful types to dilute the alcohol to a greater degree, thus reducing its potency in their systems.

It also means that if you're a woman, chances are you will be more affected by drinking than a man—even one of the same size. Whereas a typical male body is composed of about 60 percent water, the typical female body, because of smaller muscle mass, has about 55 percent water. "What this means, basically, is that women are down a couple of quarts," said Dr. O'Brien. And the deficit means the alcohol will affect females more.

Other factors besides size also affect how your body responds to alcohol. The drinking environment and your emotional state can play a significant role in this, for example. If you're upset or angry about something, or if you're uncomfortable with the crowd you're with, you'll naturally feel out of sorts—and the impact of the alcohol will be heightened.

While it's not good to mix alcohol with a bad mood, the worst thing of all to mix it with is other drugs. "The major danger is mixing alcohol with tranquilizers, such as Valium," said Dr. O'Brien. "If you take these drugs in combination, the chance of dying because your respiration stops is extremely high." This is because the chemical interaction greatly intensifies the impact of the drugs.

Mixing alcohol and cocaine is likewise extremely dangerous, Dr. O'Brien said. The cocaine is a stimulant; it makes you feel wired, and this sudden burst of alertness can mask your degree of drunkenness. So you may keep drinking—or maybe you'll think you're okay to drive. Then, when the cocaine wears off in fifteen to twenty minutes, the full impact of your intoxication comes flooding back.

Not much is absolute in life, but according to Dr. O'Brien, this is: Don't ever mix alcohol with other drugs. The combination can be deadly.

## An Acquired Tolerance

Suppose you're at a party with a couple of friends. You notice they're both drinking the same thing—say, wine coolers—at about the same pace. They each put away four in an hour and a half.

Suddenly, you're struck by the difference you see. One friend, who has had quite a bit of experience with alcohol, does not seem affected much at all. Maybe she's a little more animated than usual, or slurring a word now and then. But that's about it.

Your other friend, meanwhile, is visibly loaded. This friend has never had anything to drink before. She's acting boisterously. Her slurring is serious and her balance isn't too hot, either. Could they possibly have consumed the same amount of alcohol?

The answer is yes. And the reason is that the body is capable of developing a tolerance for alcohol. People who drink regularly aren't as affected as much by a given quantity. They show fewer visible signs of intoxication, because their bodies have become accustomed— and more resistant—to the effects of the drink. They actually may have a slightly lower blood alcohol level, too, since their bodies have become a little better at metabolizing it.

This does not mean, however, that alcohol is any less dangerous to the experienced drinker's system. The idea here is not that practice makes perfect, and that you should get in as much partying as you can so alcohol won't get to you as much. It is the same toxic drug when taken in excess, no matter how many drinks you've downed in your lifetime. Tolerance simply means that you're better at hiding the effects.

An unusual aspect to tolerance is that, in many cases, even the heaviest of drinkers will eventually lose it altogether. In advanced stages of alcoholism, many drinkers will go from being able to hold liquor by the jugful to seeming to get drunk just by whiffing it. This is believed to be the result of a heightened sensitivity of the brain, which has been damaged from the years of drinking.

## The High Toll

Even if you're the size of Mr. T, or have the highest tolerance on the block, you're going to get drunk if you drink a lot. Maybe it will take you five or six drinks, instead of the two or three it would require for a less imposing body. But you *will* get drunk. And if you have too much to drink regularly, the alcohol will slowly but steadily damage your body.

The extent of the damage varies, of course, on the extent of the drinking. But you don't need to be downing a fifth of vodka or two six-packs of beer every day for the stuff to start causing significant physical problems.

Prolonged abuse of alcohol can lead to brain damage. In the most extreme cases, the damage is irreversible. The function of your brain cells becomes impaired, and it never gets better.

This will not happen to light or moderate drinkers. But it's worth keeping in mind.

Alcohol poses other risks as well. It can increase your risk of heart disease and heart attack; stomach ulcers; mouth and throat cancer; and disorders in the pancreas. Even for the so-called weekend warrior—someone who drinks little during the week but makes up for it at the end—the down side is considerable. Elevated blood pressure, nerve damage, mental impairment, a marked increase in blood cholesterol levels—there may be this and more to deal with.

This is to say nothing of the harm from a poor diet— most heavy drinkers don't spend a lot of time worrying about getting three squares a day—or from the body's biggest trouble spot of all when it comes to alcohol: the liver.

Because the liver is the place where the alcohol gets

broken down and removed from the system, it's also the place where alcohol's harmful effects are most evident. Every time we drink too much, the liver actually is injured. Liver cells die and are replaced by scar tissue. The more frequent the alcohol abuse, the more scarring that occurs. The scarring hinders the liver's ability to function, and that isn't good, since its functions—converting foods into usable forms and producing important enzymes, among other things—are vital to good health.

Several different ailments are lumped together under the heading "alcoholic liver disease." One is a fatty liver, which is marked by a buildup of fat deposits on the liver. Another is alcoholic hepatitis, the result of the liver becoming inflamed and liver cells dying. But the most serious of all liver diseases is cirrhosis.

The word "cirrhosis" comes from the Greek term *kirrhos*, which means "orange-colored"—the color of the liver when it has this condition. Cirrhosis is characterized by serious scarring of the liver tissue, a process that breaks down the organ and leaves less of it left to function. The disease cannot be reversed and is often fatal.

## Hanging On

There's another effect of drinking, too, one that arrives much more quickly and is far more tangible.

Sharon was talking about the first time she got drunk. About how her emotions spilled out of control, about sleeping in a strange place in a stranger's house. But mostly she remembers the next day.

"I wanted to die," said Sharon. "I really did." She's not the first to wish that on the day after. Hangovers will do that to you.

What exactly is a hangover? It's what happens when

you consume too much alcohol. We talked before about alcohol being an anesthetic. If you've ever had an operation and been knocked out by an anesthetic, you may remember the blah, washed-out, disagreeable feelings that arrived the next day. You might have had a headache and nausea, too. An alcohol hangover can feature all of these symptoms and more. If you've really had a lot to drink, it will feature them in full force.

The specific symptoms vary from person to person, but generally when you're hung over you can count on a pounding headache, nausea, some dizziness, and a high sensitivity to noise and light and movement. Fatigue and depression are often part of the package, too. It is not anybody's idea of a good time.

A hangover is basically a reaction to a toxic amount of alcohol. "It stems from the adverse effect of the alcohol on the brain," said Dr. O'Brien. The alcohol increases the fluid in the brain, creates marked changes in the membranes surrounding the brain cells, and reduces those cells' ability to function. The upshot is discomfort. A lot of it.

Many people insist hangovers are brought on, or made worse, by drinking different kinds of liquor and using different kinds of fruits and mixers with that liquor.

"People say they got sick because they mixed all their drinks," said Dr. O'Brien, "but it's all a myth. People will tell me they were hung over because of all the different fruits they put in their drinks. I say, 'You have different fruits every morning, and then you say it's healthy.'

"You drink too much, you get sick. It's that simple," he said. "It's a result of the direct toxic effect of alcohol on the brain." All the theories and speculation about what drink did what, says Dr. O'Brien, "are absolute myths."

There have been hangover remedies—by the dozens—ever since there have been hangovers. Warren swears that having three or four tall glasses of water—the more the better—takes the edge off his hangovers. Others report relief from Vitamin C, fruit juice, eggs, or any number of other things. Aspirin is a popular option, too.

"There's an ad out saying that after you've been drinking you'll feel much better in the morning if you take an aspirin before you go to bed," said Dr. O'Brien. "It's one of the worst ads I've ever seen. Aspirin can cause bleeding. The alcohol has already irritated your stomach lining. Having aspirin will only foul it up some more."

Probably the most well-known hangover antidote is to have a small sampling of what you were drinking the night before. It's called having a nip of "the hair of the dog that bit you." Some people swear by it. Here, too, Dr. O'Brien isn't buying. "That will only prolong the agony and make the hangover last longer," he said. Just as in the case with breaking the alcohol down, the cure for a hangover, he said, is time.

"That's really the only solution," he said. "Your system has had a big shock. There has been tremendous central nervous system depression. If you drink too much, plan on having a hangover."

## Fun and Games?

Maggie was at a party. "I felt like shocking people," she said. "I've always had this image as Little Miss Goody Two Shoes, and I wanted to show them another side of me." With that, Maggie accepted a dare. And she downed an entire pint of Peachtree, a flavored brandy.

She succeeded in shocking people. "They couldn't believe it," Maggie said. "They were standing there, shaking my arm, saying, 'You okay? You okay?' " Maggie said she was fine. "I wasn't drunk. Just a little light-headed, that's all."

There are nearly as many ways and styles of drinking as there are drinks. Some people enjoy sipping a glass of wine. Others will down a cold beer after some strenuous work on a hot day. Some will emulate adults they've watched and have a mixed drink before dinner.

Drinking games are big, too. Maybe you've played, or seen others play, a game called quarters, in which a coin is flipped into a glass, and various participants drink, depending on whether it lands in the glass. Other people like to play word or quiz games, in which you have to take a drink if you mess up or don't know the answer.

Chugging is another popular game. In this one, the idea is to guzzle the alcohol—usually beer—as fast as you can. Sometimes people will engage in beer-drinking contests, which call for chugging one beer after another. Some people find it amusing to drink in this fashion, not least because the alcohol gets inside you so fast that the high seems instantaneous, almost as though somebody flicked a switch.

## Too Much, Too Fast

The fact is, however, that there isn't much amusing about subjecting yourself to risk. And that's exactly what a chugger is doing, particularly if he or she is chugging high-proof alcohol, as Maggie did. She consumed sixteen ounces of 96 proof alcohol. She was being playful. She wanted "to shock the socks off my friend." She could well have shocked him in another way: by dying.

"This kind of drinking is extremely dangerous," said Dr. O'Brien. "People don't realize that average lethal blood level for alcohol if you're under twenty years old is .32 percent." It's about .4 percent for those over twenty. According to Dr. O'Brien, half the people who reach such a concentration of alcohol in their bloodstream will die.

"Never, ever chug a pint," he said. If you weigh 150 pounds and you put down a pint of 80 proof alcohol, you're blood alcohol level is going to be about .32 percent. If you weigh 120 pounds, it will be .40 percent. It may seem like a fun thing to do. But this kind of fun nobody needs.

One of the reasons such levels are so dangerous is because it's very easy for your breathing to simply stop. "The respiratory system becomes so depressed it can just quit altogether," said Dr. O'Brien. "I've seen it happen time after time."

Another big danger, he says, is the heightened risk of aspiration, which is choking on your own vomit. As Dr. O'Brien explains, your system slowdown is so great that the body's reflexes to cough and vomit aren't working correctly. "You don't have your normal defenses going," he said, "so you have much more of a chance of something getting lodged in your trachea." And of choking to death.

Dr. O'Brien cautions that if you're with a friend who is extremely drunk, never leave him or her alone. Don't even let your friend go to the bathroom alone. You never know when this blockage might occur. If your friend does begin choking, quickly position the person so the head is lower than the rest of the body so as to induce the lodged particle to work free. If nothing is stuck in the throat but breathing has stopped, administer mouth-to-mouth resuscitation.

## Conflicting Signals

Alcohol can ravage the human body; we've seen ample evidence of this. And yet, its dangers can be very easy to overlook. "Somehow we put alcohol in another category from other drugs," said Dr. O'Brien. And it's plain to see why. Alcohol is legal. It's sold in thousands of different places around the country, and served in tens of thousands. Not only is it socially acceptable, for a lot of people it's practically a social obligation—the only way when it's time for fun.

Our society sends a distinct double message to us, and nobody gets it more forcefully than young people. You turn on the TV, and right after you see a "Just Say No" to drugs spot, you're liable to see Spuds McKenzie or Joe Piscopo trying to sell you beer. Over and over, in place after place, we see liquor served and people seeming to enjoy it and everything being just dandy. One study showed that the average young person will see alcohol consumed on television seventy-five-thousand times by the time he or she reaches the legal drinking age. The reinforcement is everywhere.

John Lucas is a professional basketball player who is recovering from addiction to cocaine and alcohol. He also works a lot with young people to alert them to the dangers of all kinds of drugs. "The biggest problem is this double message," he said. "You may have a parent who will say, 'Okay, you can have a graduation party. But there will be no drugs.' Then the parents will go out and buy a keg of beer.

"Alcohol is the biggest drug killer of all," said John Lucas.

Shirley is fourteen years old. The double message has reached her, very clearly. "Drugs are definitely a no," she said. "You know they can really hurt you. But alcohol is there and you see older kids doing it, and they provide it. It's there. It's everywhere."

Added Robert, "Drugs you can get addicted to. Alcohol is safer. You can continue to use it, because you're not as addicted as easily. People I know say they can stop any time. If they say that, I guess it must be easy."

"Drugs are a lot more serious. If you do drugs, you can get addicted," said Jill. "You never think drinking is going to harm you. Everyone is doing it. It's like, 'Hey, let's have a good time.' No one really thinks much about it."

Which is exactly the point. Because it is so prevalent, and so socially acceptable, alcohol gets lightweight treatment from many, many people. It's also treated this way because everybody is sure they can handle it. Alcohol problems only happen to other people.

Dennis thought that. He is a recovering alcoholic. "My drinking almost killed me," he said. "But you never think you will have a problem. You always think you will never let it get out of control."

## The Wrong Message

We're all trained to think that the stuff just isn't strong enough or serious enough or addictive enough to give us problems. We'll look at this attitude more when we hear from some teenage alcoholics a little later. For now, we just need to keep in mind that this training is wrong. Very wrong. And also very dangerous. Yes, millions of people drink without it interfering with their lives. But millions of others drink—and have it wreck their lives.

There are at least 12 million alcoholics in this country. Alcohol abuse results in nearly 100,000 deaths each year. Some 750,000 others are injured in drunken-driving accidents annually. The yearly cost of alcohol abuse, in accidents, health care costs, and lost work, is roughly $116 billion.

It's not your fault if you've gotten the double message, if your sense is, from all you've seen and heard, that alcohol is not something to be overly concerned about. It's not any individual's fault, really. It's an attitude that's all around us, that society at large hammers home.

It is why many experts consider alcohol abuse the biggest health problem in this country. And why the sooner we accept that the double message is a lie, the better off everyone's going to be.

# Chapter 3

# NO THANKS
# Teenagers' Reservations About Drinking

You hear some people talk, and you'd think liquor was a miracle in a bottle (or can). You may even have gotten that idea in Chapter 1, when we heard from people who said it increased their fun, decreased their boredom, made it easier to relate to the opposite sex, and helped in coping with problems. Others said it made them more confident, made them fit in better, helped them feel both cooler and older.

Sounds like quite an endorsement, no question. But not everyone we talked with shared those feelings. In this chapter we're going to hear from kids who used to drink but who have stopped or cut down, and also from some who have chosen not to drink at all. In many cases, these are friends and classmates of those we heard from earlier. Yet their perspectives could hardly be more different.

## Alcohol-Free Fun

Darrin is seventeen and doesn't drink. He used to, a lot. He's a recovering alcoholic, and we'll find out more about his alcohol problem a little later. But now he's talking about having fun, and how it's much easier than he thought it could be.

"I go out with friends now, go places, go dancing, and none of us are drinking," he said. "We're totally straight, and it's wild. It's a really good time. If you walked into one of these dances and you'd never seen it before, you would think everybody is toasted, the way they're acting and jumping around. But nobody is. You talk to them and they're coherent. You can understand what they're saying. Then they get up and dance and go all over the place, and they're totally straight.

"When I drank," Darrin went on, "I thought that you *had* to drink to socialize. It was like it didn't even count unless there was drinking going on. But that's all wrong. Sometimes I'd have fun when I would drink, but I also would have fights and black out and get into trouble. I have more fun now than I ever did."

Evan, too, thinks fun doesn't have to mean drinking. "Definitely not," he said. "You don't need it, and you may be able to have more fun without it. Say you're going to see an event, like a stand-up comedy show. You go when you're drunk and you're not going to understand half the things that they're talking about, and yet you laugh anyway because everybody else is. But if you're not drunk, and you actually understand it, it's going to be much funnier. You're going to have a better time."

Evan said the same is true at parties. "You can not drink and have as much or more fun as everybody who's drinking and passing out all over the place. You know what you're doing, that's why. You can understand more things going on around you."

Richard agrees totally. "People say to be happy you have to have alcohol at a party," he said. "That's not true. It makes fights. It can make people unhappy. People say they have fun, but they drink and they don't know what they're going to do, and they start making trouble with other people.

"We have fun at parties and we don't need alcohol. Why do you need it? We play around, play games and all that. Who needs it?"

## Learning by Example

Ellen has chosen not to drink. She says it's mainly because she has an alcoholic father. The drinking has played a big part in her parents' divorce. A warm, kind man when sober, Ellen's father turns nasty with alcohol inside him. Ellen wants no part of him when he's like that. And no part of drinking at all at this point in her life.

"It's just a personal decision," Ellen said. "Not that everyone who does it is bad, or gets into trouble. I'm just too afraid I'd fall into it."

Ellen will go to parties where there's drinking, but feels no urge to join in. "I like to know what's going on all the time," she said. "I don't want to do something stupid, or have someone do something stupid to me."

Jill's attitudes have been markedly affected by a parent as well. She told of being at a friend's Sweet Sixteen party where many of the guests were drinking. Without paying it much mind, Jill got caught up in it. She had a drink, then another. Then the guys mixed a bunch of different kinds of alcohol together into one potent mish-mash. "I didn't know what I was drinking," said Jill. But she drank anyway. And she got buzzed quickly.

Suddenly, Jill's thoughts turned to her father, who has had problems with drinking for years. He gets very disagreeable when drunk. "He drives crazy, he gets mad, he hits you, throws things at you," said Jill. "And now here I was drinking, and I was thinking, 'Oh my God, what am I doing?' That's what stopped me, really. I was doing what I always said I wouldn't do. I got really upset that night because of what I did."

Jill says what she has seen alcohol do to her father has made her very cautious with her drinking. It has made her mother cautious, too. "She doesn't even go near it herself," said Jill. "If I ask her for one, she'll say, 'You can have it, as long as you watch it and are careful how you drink, and that you realize that you don't need it to have fun. You already have all your friends. You don't need this at all.' That's what she'll tell me, and I think that's good. You do have to be very careful."

Jill, by the way, is one person who doesn't buy the double message we talked of earlier. "I don't see any difference between alcohol and drugs," she said. "Kids take drugs for the same reason they drink. They like the high, they want to get happy, forget about their problems. A lot of these people say alcohol is nothing, it's no big deal. But when you come right down to it, when you say this person snorts and that person shoots and another person drinks, they're doing it for the same reason. It's stupid to say drugs are bad, but that you can drink. There's no difference to me."

## "Don't Be Like Me"

As it did for Ellen and Jill, a family problem has played a big part in Ernie's feeling about alcohol. In his case the problem drinker was his older brother. "There was a lot of trouble with my brother," said Ernie, who is seventeen. "He dropped out of school and he was getting wasted all the time. He drank a lot. Once he decided to steal my mom's truck for an evening and he crashed it. He ran away with a girl who was a pot dealer. One time, after a big, big fight, my mother said to me, 'Do you see what this is doing? Do you see what it can do?' "

Ernie saw. And the message was reinforced by his brother himself. "He influenced me not to drink much," Ernie said. "He would say, 'Don't be like me. I don't want to see you drinking or smoking pot and cigarettes and doing all this stuff. It's bad for you.' "

Ernie drinks, but only in moderation. "If I get a slight buzz, that's it, then I stop," he said. "I've been around lots of messed-up people. I saw that's where my brother went wrong. He would hang out with these friends and they would give him alcohol and he thought they were great, but all they were doing was dragging him down with them. That's what my parents would always point out to me.

"It sunk in a lot," said Ernie. "I know my parents are my real friends, not somebody at a party who's saying, 'C'mon drink this or drink that.' That's why a little bit of a buzz is enough for me. That's the point of why I drink. It's to relax, that's all. I've seen the harm that it can do."

## Seeing Isn't Believing

When they think weekend, lots of people think party. Ellen has a different outlook. When she thinks weekend, she thinks about listening to kids replaying the details of their excesses.

She hears it a lot. She's baffled by it.

"On Monday mornings in school you hear about this party and that one," said Ellen. "You never hear about what people talked about or anything like that. You hear about how sick everybody got or the crazy stuff they did. Everything is party, party, party. They joke about it, saying, 'You were so funny, you acted like such a jerk.' I don't understand, and I probably never will."

Many teenagers we talked to spoke about this. They said they cut back their alcohol consumption after getting an eyeful of the wild, sometimes dangerous things that happen when booze is flowing.

Allison felt she acted pretty stupidly at a few parties. "You lose control over everything you do," she said. "You do the dumbest things." So she decided to try an experiment. She went to a party and had nothing to drink and sat back and watched the goings-on.

"I just wanted to see what would happen," Allison said. "And I saw so many stupid things, and it really hit me, that if I were drinking I would be doing those same stupid things. I mean, they start fights for the dumbest reasons. They have egg tosses in somebody's house. They're throwing them off the ceiling. People are loud and running around half naked. Just a lot of crazy things."

Allison still drinks now and then. Sometimes she even gets drunk, she says. But she says she's much more aware of what drinking can do. "I think it's bad experiences, more than anything, that make you see that," she said. "There are so many parties where you remember what you did and you regret it. You think about facing those people the next day and you're so embarrassed. You can't believe what you did. It's like, 'You mean I paraded around with no pants on?' One party, I remember I had alcohol all over my legs. I told my friend it was really burning because I had cuts there. Well, I put that alcohol on my legs. Not anybody else. I was drunk and I just took it and spread it around, just fooling around. That's the kind of stupid things you can do."

## Drinking and Daring

Jerry used to drink, but doesn't anymore. He started when he was twelve, smuggling a beer at home. He never drank vast quantities and didn't like alcohol's effect on him. "I would sneak some in the house. Sometimes I would get drunk in my room. I'd smoke cigarettes up there, and if my parents came in and asked about the smell, I'd tell them it must be something I was burning in my chemistry set. I was really bad. I did stupid things. If I ever got caught, they would've killed me." Jerry said the alcohol made him reckless. He tells of the time he had one beer and took out his brother's souped-up car and had it doing 115 miles per hour before the police (who had set up a roadblock) forced him off the road. He wasn't drunk, but it's pretty clear his one can affected his judgment. "I hated myself when I drank," he said. "I acted like a jerk."

If Jerry needed any reinforcement to stop, he got it from his friends, just as Allison did. "I saw them while I wasn't drunk a couple of times. I watched their actions. And they were making fools of themselves. And I said to myself, "Why the hell am I ruining my life by drinking?"

He has become adamantly anti-alcohol. Not just because of the powerful and negative effect it had on him, but also because he and several friends were seriously injured when a drunk smashed head on into the car they were traveling in.

"I hate drinking," says Jerry. He tells of hanging out in a courtyard in school and overhearing a couple of kids talking about a party. One of them was boasting about

7his escapades—how drunk he got, how he carried on, and so on.

"I didn't even know this kid, and I just started yelling at him. I told him how stupid that was," said Jerry. He smiled somewhat sheepishly at the memory. "I couldn't even believe I was saying it, but it just came out. Later a friend who saw what I did came up and said, 'Gee, I guess you really don't like drinking, huh?' "

Laurie is sixteen and has only had a taste of alcohol. She has no interest in having more; like Jerry, she has seen what it can do. "The main thing for me is watching other people drink. One of my friends, he was at a party, and he got drunk and didn't know who he was or where he was going, or who any of us were. He thought I was his girlfriend. It was really crazy. He made a fool out of himself.

"I've seen too many people get hurt when they get drunk," Laurie continued. "I've seen fights. I've seen people get into cars and ride around. They're so confident in themselves they think they can do anything. Their attitude is I'm 'A-1 and I can handle it. Let's go dragging down the Turnpike!' "

Laurie also has become convinced, from what she's seen, that alcohol is no problem-solver. She knows a lot of people who say they drink to get away from their problems. She sees that it does them no good. "I think a much better idea than drinking is to go for a drive," she said. "I just like getting in the car and driving when something is bothering me. It just gets you out of the house and relaxes you for a while, and you can calm down and go back and try to work on your problem again." Laurie laughed and said, "The worst you can do is run out of gas.

"But with drinking, you get drunk and then when you

sober up, the problem is there again and you're right back where you started."

## Leaving a Bad Taste

"Nasty, the stuff tastes nasty." That was Evelyn's reaction when she had her first drink at a wedding a couple of years ago. She had only a few sips that day, just a bit of beer, wine, and champagne. It was enough to know she thought alcohol tasted pretty awful.

"I tasted it and I just thought it was disgusting," she said. "I don't know what people like in it."

Evelyn is fourteen and in the eighth grade. She doesn't drink, mostly because of her feeling about the taste, but partly because of what happens after it's consumed. "I'd never want to drink," she said. "I'd feel weird. Alcohol does a lot of weird things that I wouldn't want to do."

Mary is no fan of the taste, either. Her first drinking experience came at age twelve. It was whiskey. She won't soon forget it. "At a fiftieth anniversary celebration at my church this lady asked my mother if it would be okay for me to have a little sip of something," Mary said. "My mom said, 'Okay, why not? Just a little bit.' But that was no little bit she gave me. I took some and it turned my stomach."

Suddenly Mary felt nauseous. It made her scared. The feeling kept getting worse. She told her mother how bad she felt. And off they went to the emergency room.

"I wasn't there but half a minute and I threw up," said Mary. "It may taste good to some people, but your body hates it. Your body won't accept it."

Mary stays a long way from whiskey. She limits her alcohol intake to special occasions and then will only sip minute amounts of champagne. That's the one drink she thinks isn't vile.

"I hate the taste, too," said Jerry. "I used to smoke a couple of cigarettes before I would drink. That would make it so I wouldn't taste it as much and could get it down."

## Regrettable Developments

Sharon was at a party. She had a beer, then another. And another. And a few after that. Except for one slice of pizza, her stomach had been empty. Sharon got hammered.

"At first I was hyper, really hyper," she said. "I was running all around, and when people tried to help me, I would yell, 'Leave me alone.' Then I started crying. I heard the cops were coming to the party, and I started crying and I just couldn't stop. I was scared."

Much of the night remains a blur. Sharon does remember sleeping on the floor somewhere—and that her stomach soon began its revolt. She slept for a while, then raced for the bathroom. She threw up, went back to sleep, then threw up again. So it went all night.

Sharon awoke the next morning. "I didn't have a headache," she said. "But I just kept throwing up. My stomach was what killed me. I felt like never drinking again. I'd been drunk before this, sometimes a lot, and I'd never gotten this sick. I felt like dying."

Alcohol was a long way from a miracle in a bottle for Sharon. "I would never drink that much again," she said.

Harry is fifteen. He stopped drinking because he felt he was heading for trouble. He drank a lot, Friday night to Sunday night, for about a year and a half. Fistfights at the local hangout, brushes with police, and vandalism became regular occurrences. But the clincher came one night when he simply asked if he could go to the movies and his father said no. Harry went out with his friends. He got drunk. He came back to the house and smashed the windows of his father's car.

"I was grounded for three months," Harry said. "It just made me think, 'If this is what's going to happen, then screw it, it's not worth it.'"

Lisa never had the acute troubles Harry did. But she'd been drinking for several years, and she began noticing that it was getting harder to stop. It scared her.

"I remember one time at this party, I vowed I was only going to have one," she said. "I promised myself that. I was sure I could do it. Well, I had the one, and I said, 'Well, one more isn't going to hurt, just this one.' And before I knew it I'd had like eleven."

Lisa realized she wanted alcohol far more than she had known. There was no way around it, she thought: She was getting hooked. And that was what she needed to make her decide to get unhooked. Lisa is sixteen, and doesn't drink at all anymore.

## The Parent Factor

Richard has a very close relationship with his parents. He respects them, and what they say, very much. "My father has explained to me the problems you can have with drinking," Richard said. "He told me how people use it to escape their problems, and how much harm drinking can cause." Richard has had a glass of wine at home, but that's about it.

"My father has said that it's best if I don't drink now, not at this age." Richard is thirteen. This is plenty of reason to lay off liquor. It hasn't always been easy.

Richard told of a time in fifth grade when he was coming home from school with a friend. "A close friend," said Richard. "We were walking through the woods and he pulled out this bottle of wine. He was all excited. He said it was strong and very sweet. He just kept trying to tempt me. He'd say, 'Oh man, your mother's not here. We could have fun. After you drink some of this, nothing will matter. I've got candy here. We're alone. We'll have a blast. Your mom ain't gonna know.'"

Richard kept resisting. His friend stayed after him, kept urging him, telling him not to be such a baby. Finally, Richard just bolted. "I started running and I kept running. I ran right out of the woods. I dropped a book along the way and I never found it. Later I had to pay for it." For Richard it was worth the price. He didn't want to drink—and he stuck to what he wanted.

Why did Richard feel so strongly about it? "I didn't have my parents' permission to drink," he said. "Plus back then I didn't really know what it was going to do to me if I drank. I really didn't know anything about alcohol." Richard said he figured he'd lost a friend because of the incident. But the next day, his friend approached him. "He said he was sorry. I said, 'That's okay, just don't do it to me again.' We're still friends."

## Showing the Way

Leslie is very cautious about her drinking for a different reason. She has a little sister who is nine. "I really want to set a good example for her," Leslie said.

"Sometimes it's really hard. It's hard to put your life aside, your problems aside, so you don't demonstrate something bad to your younger sibling. There have been times I've said I've had enough and wanted to run away. I even left a few times, but now I can't do that, because my sister is older and I don't want her to think that the way to deal with a problem is to run away.

"It's the same thing with drinking," Leslie went on. "My sister doesn't understand the anger or the pressures I may feel, but God, if she ever saw me pull out a bottle, then she would pick up on that after a while and think that's how I deal with things so it must be all right. I know she's seen it on TV, because it's everywhere on TV. Then she would see it at home, too? She would have to think, 'It's okay to do that.'"

Leslie is eighteen, and drinks "a couple of times a month." She looks back now and wishes she hadn't started. She says she'll try to help her sister wait until she's legal age to drink.

"If I had waited, I would've been much better off than I am now," said Leslie. "I think I would've felt better about myself. I would've saved myself until I was twenty-one. My self-respect would've been higher if I had waited, because then I wouldn't have been driven into it. Instead of following everybody's lead at parties, I wished I would've said no, no. It would've made me feel better, stronger, knowing I didn't just go along, and that I dealt with my problems on my own.

"I think what I'll tell my sister is that I'm always there for you. If you need help with anything, I'm there. Don't turn to alcohol and drugs. Turn to me. Alcohol and drugs may help temporarily, but that's it. Your problems will remain."

# Chapter 4

## THE HOME FRONT
## Talking to Parents About Drinking

Sally opened the door and her body tensed up with anxiety. "I was really afraid they would notice," she said. "I thought they would be able to tell there was something different about me."

She had just returned home from a party. Sally was thirteen, and had gotten drunk for the first time. "Everybody was drinking, and they offered me some and all my friends were saying, 'Yeah, yeah.' So I figured I might as well take some also." She became giggly and animated. "I wasn't walking too straight, either," said Sally.

She had fun. Time went fast. Then the party ended and she had to go home. Suddenly the fear starting welling up inside her. Reality slammed into Sally's gut. She had to face her parents. She composed herself and put on the soberest front possible as she walked carefully into the house.

66

"I said I was really tired and I went straight to bed," said Sally. "They looked at me as if I were different, but they never said anything about it. They wondered why I was home a bit later than usual and I made up some excuse, which they believed."

"They never questioned me," Sally said. And if they had found out? "I would've been in real big trouble."

## Concealing the Evidence

If you've ever had anything to drink, chances are you've either faced a variation of the same dilemma or done everything in your power to avoid facing it. Maybe you've come home buzzed or drunk, too. Maybe you've told your parents you were going to Activity A, when you were really going to Activity B—to drink. Maybe you've called them up and told them you were sleeping over at a friend's house; you don't tell them it's because you're pretty far gone and you would prefer they not know. Or maybe you've had to call for a ride because you were too drunk to drive, or got nailed at a school function for drinking a beer behind the gym and had the principal summon your parents in for a conference.

For a lot of people, dealing with their parents about alcohol is one of the toughest things of all. In this chapter, we're going to hear from your peers about what they feel parents should and shouldn't do; about leveling with parents as well as lying to them; about how some parents handle the issue of drinking well and how others really mess it up; and how teens would handle things if they were doing the parenting.

## Heavy-Handed Treatment

Talking about drinking with her parents would be constructive, says Laurie. In fact, she would welcome it. The subject does come up, but Laurie says the exchange is a long way from constructive.

"We don't have family discussions," Laurie said. "It's more like my Mom saying, 'If you ever get drunk, I'll kill you.' Then my father will come in two minutes later and he'll say, 'Laur, if I ever find you drunk at a party, you'll never live to see your next birthday.' "

The approach bothers Laurie. "I mean, they don't sit down and talk to me about it. They never have, not once. They just seem to yell and scream at me, because they don't want me to get drunk."

The results of the bellowing? "It goes in one ear and out the other," Laurie said. "I can't stand people yelling at me. I listen better when people talk to me, rather than nagging me every two minutes of the day. Every time I get in trouble, the first thing my parents say is, 'Are you drunk? Are you on drugs?' "

Laurie says she has had a total of half a can of beer in her life. She also says it has nothing to do with her parents' badgering, but everything to do with her friends. "I see what they do at parties, when they get drunk, and it really gets out of hand."

Karen's parents used a similarly heavy-handed approach to the subject. "When I was younger," said Karen, "my father said to me, 'If you ever smoke, take drugs, or drink, I'm going to break your fingers so you won't be able to pick anything up.' "

"My parents don't trust me at all," said Karen. "I'm not allowed to go out with my friends. They're afraid I'll go out to a party instead. I can't tell my parents anything."

Jerry is sixteen. He says sermons from his parents were standard fare at his house when he was a little younger. "Every time I walked out the door I would get a lecture about drinking," he said. "Every time. They'd say, 'Is there going to be any alcohol at this party?' " The lectures must be pretty common; as Jerry spoke, a tableful of teenagers nodded in agreement.

## Diminishing Returns

Jerry doesn't drink anymore. He used to, but as we've seen, it had a very powerful effect on him, so he stopped. He thinks one of the reasons he drank was because of his parents' preaching to him. He didn't care for it—and drinking was a way of getting back at them.

Karl didn't like the way his parents handled his drinking, either. "I felt like they were talking down to me, treating me like a little kid, telling me what I have to do, what I can't do," he said. When they come on too strong that way, Karl said, "It would make me put up a front and go against what they say. Sometimes I just want to drink to spite them."

Weslie agrees. "My mother doesn't trust me. She doesn't trust that I can make decisions for myself. She gets on me a lot. If you have a fight with your mom, you go out to drink to forget about it, and because you know it's wrong and you do it to get back at her."

Time and again, we heard talk about how counterproductive it was for parents to threaten or badger kids about drinking. Virtually everyone said it only increases the teenager's urge to rebel. And it wasn't just kids who wanted their parents to be more lenient and understanding about teenage drinking who felt this way. Jerry, for instance, believes it's better for parents to be stricter than his were with him.

"They would hardly ever punish me for anything," he said. "And even when they did, they usually wouldn't stick to it for very long." Jerry has no problem with parents taking a strong stand on drinking. But he does have a problem when his parents, rather than explaining why they feel it important for him to abstain, harass him with questions and threats.

"I think preaching is one of the worst things you can do," said Randi. "I won't preach to my kids. I want to explain things to them. I'll want my child to know what alcohol can do and to expose the glamor behind it, and show how it's a gimmick. But you have to do it without preaching."

## Attitude Adjustments

For Ernie, parents' attitudes in talking to you make all the difference. "A lot of kids rebel because their parents treat them like kids. They say, 'Don't do it,' and then the kids will ask why, and they say, 'Because I said so.' Parents often don't give reasons. They don't talk to their kids. They just say, 'I'm the parent and that's that.'" Many others agreed that when you get the because-I-said-so routine, you feel like you're being bullied. And that doesn't make you very receptive to the message.

"It's much better when your parents put you on the same level, treat you like a human, not a little pet, you know, don't do this, don't do that," Ernie said. "A kid will have a lot more respect for his parents and he will be more prone to listen to them, and think about what they're saying. I think the biggest thing is for parents to trust the kids."

Karl has begun to notice a change in his parents, and he likes it. They used to be on his case about drinking all the time. "But we sat down a couple of weeks ago and I felt that for the first time they were treating me almost like an equal. They weren't looking down to me, telling me what I have to do. We talked seriously. My mother said something like, 'I don't mind that much if you have a beer or two, as long as you never drive and that you understand how drinking can be dangerous.'"

When your parents talk to you in this way, you get a sense of trust, and a sense that they have a higher regard for your judgment. One person after another spoke of how important these feelings are.

"I think my mother trusted that I would make the right choice about drinking," said Ellen, who has chosen not to drink. The trust made Ellen feel good—and made her relationship with her mother better.

## Building Bridges

Leslie was speaking of how supportive her parents are. "My family trusts me; I can say that right out," she said. "My mother always tells me, 'I love you, I trust you.'" Ernie heard this, and he said, "I think you really take those words into consideration when you're going out. You're just about to drink and you hear those words, 'I trust you' and it makes you feel bad if you go ahead and drink. It makes you want to show them they were right to trust you. On the other hand, if the last thing you hear before you go out is, 'If I find out you were drinking, you'll be in serious trouble,' then you're going to say, 'Ha, ha, I'm doing it,' and slug down a beer."

Honesty and trust can greatly help matters. Even those who said they lie to their parents about their drinking felt this way. They said they lie because they feel like they have to, that it's easier, that their parents would overreact or punish them severely if they didn't. Almost all of them said they don't want to lie.

"If you can be honest, it's so much easier," said Allison. "When I tell my mother the truth—and I usually do—I feel a lot better. When you talk, you get close. And when I'm close to her, I don't want to do something that will hurt her. I don't want to make her worry. I don't want to put her through that." Allison paused and added, "The biggest guilt trip in the world is when you lie to your mother."

Karen seeks openness, too. "I'd like to tell my parents what I'm doing and be open with them. But I can't do it, because they're so strict. I'm not allowed to do anything. I think if you could talk to your parents, you wouldn't drink nearly as much."

Rita smiled and looked a little ashamed as she talked about the untruths she tells her parents. "Sometimes you don't want to lie," she said. "I wish I didn't have to. I wish I didn't have to say I'm going to the movies or I'm going to peewee golf when I'm really going to a party. One time my father said to me, 'Rita, you must be a pretty good golfer.' Another time he said, 'Say, how many movies have you seen this summer?' "

She went on. "They don't trust me. Even when I tell them the truth, they don't. My mother won't believe me and we'll get in a big fight. That's not good, for your own mother not to trust you." Rita feels angry about not being trusted, and this in turn fuels her urge not to tell the truth. It's a way of evening the score.

She is convinced a better relationship with her parents would cut down on her partying. "If you're close to them, you know you would be really hurting them and disappointing them if you went out and drank, so I don't think you would. If you don't really care what they think, you'll probably go out and do it and say, 'Who cares?' I know when I'm really getting along with my mother, I am definitely more careful. I don't want to drink much or get in trouble. I'd feel really guilty if I went out and got drunk when we're getting along."

## Taking Lies Lying Down

Just about everyone we talked to thought lying to their parents was bad. Jane was an exception. She said, "I lie to my parents all the time. I just say I'm going over to a friend's house, and then we'll drink. They think I'm totally straight. I think they would be amazed and shocked if they knew what went on." Jane said it didn't bother her to lie, because if she told the truth, "they wouldn't trust me at all, and then they would take away the freedom that they give me now. Like, they don't want me going out with guys in cars. But I do. If they found out they would be mad."

One time when Jane went out riding with a guy, the guy was drunk and driving fast. There were four people in the front seat. Jane was on somebody's lap. "He drives really crazy," she said. He speeded toward an intersection, didn't see a light in time, and ran a red. They smashed into another car. "I almost went through the windshield," Jane said. "It was bad. I was really scared." She also was really scared her parents would find out how she had spent her day. They never did.

## The (Fabricated) Plot Thickens

Jane seemed as unfazed about the accident as she is about the lying. But virtually everyone else talked about lying catching up to you. They talked about how it can make you feel crummy because you know it's wrong. They talked about the distance it creates, and also about the remorse—the pangs of conscience that arrive seconds after you look squarely at your parents and tell them a large fish story. Many also said the deception is more trouble than it's worth, since you have to be concerned with making up a good alibi, getting people to cover for you, and being sure everybody involved has the same story. All this can be very stressful—not least because the more untruths you concoct, the better your chance at getting caught. Before you know it, a once-small fib about having a long play rehearsal (when you were really into a long night of drinking) spills over into elaborate tales about dead batteries, traffic jams, altered plans, the play director getting sick, and on and on.

Said Allison, "You lie about one thing and then you realize you have to lie about something else to be consistent. It gets complicated. It's just much better and easier to tell the truth."

Sharon went to a party and got drunk, and made up some story about where she was going. "My mother found out about it three weeks later. I thought I had gotten away with it. I think she talked to a friend's mother and my friend was at the party, so my mother found out that it was pretty wild and the cops were there and everything. I felt really bad, really guilty. I was grounded for about two weeks. If she had told my father, forget it. He would've killed me. One time I went over to this guy's house and they had told me not to go there. I made up something. He found out and grounded me for a month. He hates lying."

Others agreed with Sharon that their parents would be more upset about being lied to than just about anything else. Tom's mother, one of the parents we talked to, confirmed this. "I know what it's like to be young," she said. "I know what can happen, and that you can get in some tight spots. My kids drink. I tell them that if they do that, they should never, ever drive, or get in the car with somebody who has been drinking. Just call me, no matter when or where, and I'll get you. I also let them know that the one thing I absolutely demand is that they be honest with me. That's the key to everything. When you're honest, you may have disagreements, but you can work things out. Lying is the one thing I won't tolerate. I think because they know that I try to be understanding, that they really don't want to lie to me."

Said Sharon, "I kept thinking I should've told them I went to that party. I don't think my Mom would have been as mad. She would've felt better because I had been honest with her. I probably still would've been grounded, but I would've felt better about things—and they would've felt much better, too—instead of hearing it from some-body else."

## The Straight Story

Weslie spoke of a very practical side of the issue. "If I was a parent I wouldn't want my kid lying to me," she said. "I think lying is really bad sometimes. Suppose my daughter lies to me, says she's going to the movies when she's going to a party. Then she gets in trouble and needs a ride or something. She wants to call up, but feels like she can't because of the lie. And then what would happen if I got a call in the middle of the night from the hospital or the police?"

Evan said he used to lie to his father about his drink-ing. He just figured it was the easiest way to go. But then Evan's drinking got worse. He started getting drunker and drunker, more often. He was getting into trouble and he was getting worried. He could feel himself getting tugged to the bottle. He needed help, needed to talk about it. He went to his father.

"It was one of the best things I ever did," said Evan. "He was upset I was drinking in the first place, but we had a really good talk and he felt good that I was able to come to him like that. I regret any lying I did to my father. If I had known he would have understood everything and that I could really talk to him, I wouldn't have lied in the first place. When I go to confession in church, I'm still sorry for those lies, because he trusted me and I let him down."

## A Clear Message

Miguel's parents never talked to him about drinking, he said. Not really. Not in any depth. "The only time it was discussed is when my mother caught my brother when he came home one night and kissed her good night and she smelled liquor on his breath. She was talking on the phone and she told the woman to hold on, and then she said to my brother, 'If I ever catch you drinking again, I'll beat you.' "

Miguel wishes he had heard more about drinking. "Yeah, that would be really nice. It would show they care. They could explain things and tell us not to do these things. I know they care, but it's still good to talk about things like this."

Many others voiced similar opinions, saying their parents said very little, in some cases, nothing, to them about what alcohol is and what it can do.

"With my father," said Stan, "he would say, 'I don't want you drinking and driving,' but he'd never say anything about drinking itself. It was like the drinking was okay as long as I didn't get caught, or didn't drive. I think this is a very unclear message."

Evan got much the same thing from his parents. "They mentioned things here and there, but nothing much. The big thing was how dumb it was to drink and drive. They'd say stuff like that. But other than that, mostly what I heard about was drugs, not alcohol."

"There are so many people whose parents don't say anything until the kids are already drinking," said Maggie. "Then the parents object when they find out there's a party and there might be alcohol there. Then it's like, 'I've been doing this for the past three years and you haven't known about it and you're telling me now? Why didn't you mention it back when it was first being introduced?'

"Personally, I think my parents should have talked to me about it," Maggie went on. "Granted, I'm not an alcoholic or anything, but the fact is they should have said something. And that's part of the problem. A lot of kids don't really know what alcohol does. The best place to get that information is from your parents."

Maggie said if she were a parent, she would be as open as possible about it. "I'd rather have them see it in my light, instead of picking it up from kids on the bus or from TV, and start thinking having a butt and a beer is the thing to do," she said. "I would explain all about it and say, 'I want you to know drinking is bad for you, even though it's done by a lot of people and is widely accepted.' I would tell them, 'I would really prefer you not drink until you're of legal age.' I would talk to them about how bad it is to overdo it and get drunk. But I would also say, 'If you ever get in a jam, I'm here. If you need me, you have someplace to turn.' But the whole key is that they would learn from me, learn moderation."

Maggie said she was at a friend's house for New Year's once. "Her parents were really good about it," she said. "They know their kids drink, and they set an example. They called my parents and asked if it was okay if they gave me a little champagne. They said they would be there chaperoning and nobody would get ripped. But the main thing is these parents were exposing us to drinking and showing us how to drink in moderation. Which is a lot better than not talking about it, or just saying, 'I don't want you to drink and that's all.' "

## The Parents' Dilemma

It's not easy being a parent, particularly a teenager's parent. Most of the group seemed to appreciate this, and seemed to sense the conflicting thoughts some parents have: on one hand, realizing what it's like to be young and to want to experiment, and knowing drinking is very often a part of these things; and on the other hand, wanting to protect your kid, help him or her avoid trouble, make sure they don't repeat any foolish mistakes the parent may have made. A number of the teenagers said they felt their parents wanted to avoid this tension and duck the issue altogether. Which, of course, doesn't make it go away.

"You can't be naive if you're a parent," said Allison. "You can't pretend your kids aren't doing anything. These are the teenage years. A parent can't say, 'Oh, my son or daughter would never do that,' because the more you hide it or deny it, the worse it gets. It's good to talk about it. I can be very open with my mother. I can say, 'Mom, I'm going to a party tonight.' And she'll say, 'Well, be very careful, and if you need help or a ride, be sure to call.' Usually we make up that I'll call my older sister, because my father would go crazy. I can't tell *him* where I'm going or what I'm doing. I have to lie to him. My father is in the wrong. It'll work better when you're open with your children."

Leslie agrees. "You can't pretend it's not happening," she said. "A lot of parents realize their kid was drinking only after they die. They say, 'If only I hadn't pretended, if only I had faced it.' You hear those stories all the time."

## The Next Generation

Leslie drinks about twice a month. She says she has gotten drunk maybe three or four times in the past year. She thinks it's important for parents to do more than simply issue a no-drinking order to their kids. Yet Leslie says she would not want her kids to drink until they're of legal age, if at all.

"I don't think kids should be exposed to it," she said. "It's like saying that drinking is okay, and then down the line if the kid has a problem with it, the kid will say, 'Well, it was always all right at home.'

"I would try to be very honest about it. I'd try to give examples and say, 'Don't be like this person.' I wouldn't talk down to them, but I would show them how drinking is wrong and how it can waste your life. I would say, 'If you need anything, I'm here. Just don't turn to drugs or alcohol.'" As Leslie said earlier, she regrets that she drank before being of age herself.

Karl drinks quite a bit and enjoys getting drunk. But he, too, wouldn't want his kids to follow his lead. "What I would tell them is, 'What I did in high school wasn't right. I know I was wrong, and I'm telling you I made a big mistake so you won't repeat it.'" His drinking has caused problems with his own parents. And if he were a parent and his kids were going out?

"I would say, 'Just think about what you're doing. Just be sensible. I know you're smart. Don't let it get out of hand. Have a few beers if you want, be sociable, be reasonable. Have what you can handle and stop there.' And if they have a problem or can't handle it, I would say, 'Call me and I'll come and get you. If you have a problem, we'll talk about it and deal with it. We'll try to stop it from happening.' "

Evan also said he would urge his kids to refuse it. He said he would talk to them about alcohol, explain it. "And then I'd say why I think it's best not to. It gets you in trouble. I'd say, 'Do your best to refuse it. If people ask you or pressure you, all you have to do is say no. If they keep bugging you, you just keep saying no. It's only a word. Nobody's going to beat you up for it.' " The only time he would approve of teenage drinking, Evan said, was a special occasion, such as a wedding. "And I mean a drink, not getting drunk," he said.

Most of those we talked to felt their parents would be shocked if they knew the extent of the drinking that goes on. Said Allison, "If my daughter had done half the stuff I've done in the last year, I don't think I would ever let her do anything." Allison laughed. She also said she would urge her children to drink only in small amounts. She added that it would be crucial that her daughter be totally honest with her. About drinking, and everything else.

## Opening Up

This was the point the discussion kept coming back to. Teenagers with all different views on the subject of drinking—those who don't drink and those who drink a lot—felt the most vital point of all was having a dialogue. Coming to an understanding with their parents. Getting it out in the open, and getting away from lies and lectures and parental proclamations: Don't do it because I said so.

Randi said she would talk to her child at elementary school age. She summed things up well: "You want to make sure your kid can talk to you. I think it's very important for kids to trust their parents and feel like they can talk to their parents." Randi spoke about how this sense of trust and caring nurtures the child, makes him feel important, and makes his concerns and problems seem manageable.

"I want my children to have a good self-esteem, so they won't have to give in so easily to pressure," Randi said. "They won't be so affected by their peers. I never talked about my feelings. My mother worked a lot and my stepfather taught me to stuff everything inside. I just shied away from talking." Randi bottled things up. She had problems she didn't know how to deal with, or who to go to with. And the way she eventually got unbottled up was by hitting the bottle. Randi became an alcoholic.

"I'm starting to talk to my mom now," said Randi. "It's hard, but it's getting easier. Talking is very important. I open up and she opens up, and then it's both of us sharing. It's very important for a child and parent to do that."

# Chapter 5

# GETTING YOUR FILL (AND MORE)
## Talking About Getting Drunk

A warm, happy glow washes over you. Your cheeks tingle. You're relaxed, a little lightheaded, and fun comes easily. Worries? Not now. Problems? Catch me later.

You finish one, and you say, what the heck, I'll have another. And then another follows that. And pretty soon, you're more than relaxed and loose and contented. Pretty soon you're drunk.

For many young people we spoke to, getting drunk was a fairly regular occurrence. In fact, to some, getting drunk was precisely the point.

"I think that's why most kids drink," said Rita. "To get drunk. I don't mean totally bombed, or incoherent. I just mean, you know, drunk. Happy."

To others, getting drunk seems practically a rite of teenage passage. The party Friday night means getting blasted. Graduation means rolling out the keg. The big football victory means drinking some for the Gipper. Let's take a closer look at having too much to drink: at what your peers think about it, about how it feels, and about what can happen when it occurs.

## Party Time

"Practically nobody goes to a party to sip on a beer for two hours," said Allison. "You don't really think of wanting to get drunk, but you find out so and so's throwing a party Friday night, and you start drinking, and it just happens." She likes when it happens. "It's fun when you're drunk. You do the same things you would do normally; you just act a little more ridiculous than when you're sober."

Good times await when you're drunk: We heard this many times, from many different people. Your guard is lowered and you feel looser. You have a lightness of spirit. "It just makes you feel better for that time," said Sally. "You don't worry about things or worry about what other people are saying."

Miguel is eighteen. He drinks about twice a month. He has gotten drunk only a few times. He has enjoyed it. "It's wild," he said. "It feels good. It was relaxing and we did a lot of playing around. The last time, I wasn't even thinking about it. I was just having a good time, dancing, talking to the guys at this party. I didn't drink fast, but I just ended up getting drunk.

"When people get drunk they look foolish, the way they act. They fall. They look funny. They hang onto a wall and wait there for a couple of minutes. It makes me laugh. So when it happens to me, I laugh at myself and don't mind it. Like at this party, I did something really stupid. It was the end of the night. There was this neon sign hanging from the ceiling and there was a cord right by it. I thought, 'What's this?' and I unplugged it. And suddenly the music stopped. Everybody stopped and turned toward me, and there I was standing there with the cord in my hand. They looked at me and I said, 'Oh my God.' I plugged it back in and walked away."

Miguel says he usually just likes to get buzzed, except at parties. "There I like to go a little crazy," he said. But not as crazy as some, he added. After the plug episode, he went for a walk and saw one guy bending over here, getting sick, another fellow bending over there, doing the same thing. "That's really crazy," he said, "drinking so much that you get sick."

## The Flip Side

Miguel and others spoke of the euphoria of being drunk. But there is another side here, too, and that is when alcohol doesn't make for much euphoria at all. Those are the nights when having enough to drink becomes too much, when things feel out of control and the head spins and the room does likewise. Your mind gets muddled. Your tongue gets tied. And depression just descends on you, barging in out of nowhere. Lots of the teenagers we spoke to talked about these things, too.

The strength of both reactions is not surprising. Getting drunk is a powerful experience, physically and emotionally. You get drunk, you're overdosing on a drug. The results are bound to be dramatic. And sometimes, traumatic.

## On Your Way

What exactly is drunkenness? How do you know you're drunk in the first place?

"I know when I'm drunk because usually I can't walk," said Sharon. "I usually can talk, but I can't talk straight. I just sort of get mellow."

Said Joyce, "You seem a little depressed, but then something happens and you begin to overexaggerate. Somebody says something stupid and suddenly it becomes the funniest thing in the world. People look at you and say 'What are you laughing about? That's a stupid joke!' But you can't help yourself, which isn't that thrilling sometimes."

Karl knows he's drunk when he begins to lose his sense of control. "It's when I feel clumsy," he said. "I know I have a buzz when I can't walk and I'm stumbling and I'm sort of not making sense when I'm talking, stuff like that. Or if I get angry verbally, or want to lash out at somebody, then I know I've gotten a buzz. After that I know I'm drunk. Then I just want to go to sleep."

"Drunk means lying down, the bed's moving, the house is moving. You can't walk straight," said Martin.

## Sneaking Up

The word "drunk" has a severe sound to it. And the prevailing attitude seems to be that to be drunk, you need to be in quite a severe state: reeling or semiconscious, pretty much out of physical and mental control. To most of those we talked to, anything short of that qualifies only as getting buzzed or high. Sally, for instance, told of getting into a fight with her boyfriend.

She was down about it, so she invited some friends over and they all drank. "Not to the point of not knowing what I was doing," she said. "Just to get a buzz and feel better."

The physiological fact, however, is that drunkenness hits us long before the room spins or the stomach retches. And quite a bit before we don't know what we're doing. As we've seen, intoxication is measured by the amount of alcohol in the blood. And when we have .10 percent alcohol inside us, we're legally drunk. This level is reached, remember, when a 150-pound person has about four twelve-ounce beers. Karl, talking about one of his drinking escapades, spoke of a time when he had ten beers. He described himself as "a little buzzed." No matter how high your tolerance may be, you don't have that many and get a little buzzed, unless you're considerably larger than the average pro football lineman. Say, 300 pounds. And all muscle.

Karl's not quite that large, but his reaction isn't unusual, and that's because alcohol sneaks up on you. We've seen how slowly it's burned off, and how it works on the brain to lower inhibitions and hinder judgment. The result is that we tend to get a very inaccurate notion of when we're sober and when we're drunk.

The distinction is a very important one to make: not only because getting drunk regularly can do damage to the body, but also because, if you're so sure you're fine, you're going to be much more inclined to do things you shouldn't do with alcohol in you. Maybe try a dangerous stunt. Or maybe drive a car. These are simple acts, simple alcohol-induced misjudgments. And they've resulted in hundreds of thousands of injuries and deaths since people first took to the bottle.

# Buzzed, Bombed, and Beyond

After a drink or two, most people feel relaxed. They're more sociable, probably more talkative, less wound up about things. If you continue drinking, you get considerably more animated and vocal, maybe sillier, and you generally show less control over your behavior. You may not detect it, but your reactions are already slowed and your coordination is impaired.

And if you keep going from there? You start getting disoriented. You get sloppy. Your speech is slurred, you're staggering noticeably, and your emotions, by this point, may be totally out of control. You don't know what will set you off, or in what direction. Maybe you'll get very sad and start crying, or get very angry and want to sock anything that moves. Or you might swing from one emotion to another, as Donna did. She was drinking with a friend. Drinking quite a bit. "I was having a good time," she said. "I was happy, and we kept drinking, and then I got depressed. It came on fast. I just started thinking of everything I did wrong in my whole life. It started and I couldn't stop it. I was crying. I went through every single depressed time in my life."

Next arrives a virtual stupor. Your incoherence is nearly total now. You can barely talk or think. Walking? Forget it; just standing up is a major achievement. Your blood alcohol level, at this point, could well be .20 or higher, which means you're saturated with alcohol and getting dangerously close to the final stage of intoxication, which is passing out. That's the point where alcohol has depressed your system to such an extent that you become unconscious. When this occurs, you're also dangerously close, and perhaps over, the .32 level Dr. O'Brien talked about in Chapter 2—the level above which you stand a fifty-fifty chance of dying.

"With all the people who talk about how much they can drink," says Dr. O'Brien, "how come we never hear of anyone reaching a blood alcohol level of .50 percent, or .60 percent, or .70 percent? It's because you die first." The point is not that at .32 percent alcohol in your system, death is always imminent. It is that, at this level, you are a long way from just having fun or feeling relaxed or being the life of the party. You are messing with your life.

Some people who pass out just stay that way and wind up sleeping it off. Others who pass out don't wake up. Ever.

Dr. O'Brien told of a college student who had been drinking heavily at a big bash. Finally, he passed out, and his friends carted him up to his room and put him in bed. Which is where they found him, dead, the next morning.

"In almost every case like this—and I see a lot of them—the cause of death is respiratory failure," said Dr. O'Brien. The respiratory system gets so depressed that it finally quits altogether. One of the most dangerous myths about getting drunk, he says, is that if you really go too far, you'll just pass out and that's the worst of it. It would be nice if it were that tidy. Dr. O'Brien strongly advises never leaving someone who is close to passing out. Stay with him. Keep an eye an him. And make sure he doesn't have anything else to drink.

He may just stay in his stupor. But he also may pass out and then stop breathing, and if you're not around to do mouth-to-mouth resuscitation, that's the end.

## Overdoing It

Jane is about to enter high school. She drinks regularly and enjoys getting drunk. She talked about one of her recent drinking episodes, in which she was at a friend's house with some girlfriends and some older guys. "I was just laughing, going crazy," she said. There was lots of silliness and laughing and cavorting around. "I was giddy. Really hyper. I wasn't even myself. I don't even remember half of what we did. We were just doing everything and laughing, and then I thought that maybe the guys thought I was a jerk. But they didn't think that, because they understood I was drunk."

Later that day, as the drinking wore on, Jane said she got seriously drunk. "I was falling all over the place," she said. She had a drunken friend almost get run over. She got sick and had a headache and wound up getting sexually involved with a guy who was going out with someone else, and losing a friendship because of it. She also had a fight with the guy about their encounter not long after. That friendship is history, too.

Still, Jane insisted it was fun. She said, "I'll probably do it again. I know I will. I am just starting high school, and I have an older brother who will take me to all the parties."

Jane was cavalier about the whole thing. Like a few others we spoke to, she views getting drunk much more as good, wild entertainment than anything to be taken seriously. "People don't really worry about drinking," she said. "You hear about drinking and driving, but that's it. Other than that, you just always hear, 'No drugs, no drugs.' Alcohol is always there. It's just to have a good time. Nobody really has any problems with it."

Karl also was talking about getting drunk. "When do I

stop drinking?" he asked, repeating a question. "When we're out of beer or when I'm passed out. That's usually when I stop." His tone, too, was very matter-of-fact.

## Post-Prom Bomb

Tom told of the time he went to a prom and invited his date back to the house, along with a few friends. "I didn't have much in me at that point, maybe one beer," he said. Out came a bottle of Captain Morgan's Rum. "A nice big bottle," Tom said. It was half full. His friend Johnny said to him, "I bet you can't chug that."

Tom said he has a very high tolerance for alcohol. "A friend and I have drunk a case and a half of Coors and we're still standing," he said. Tom picked up the bottle and opened his throat, and down it went, every last drop.

"I said, 'Put your money on the table, Johnny,' " Tom recalled. Shortly after, Tom and his date went to leave. "I was fine," Tom said. So fine, in fact, that he was going to drive. They got in the car. "And that's the last thing I remember," said Tom. "I woke up the next morning face down on my pillow."

Tom happens to be a big, strong young man. He's the quarterback of his high school football team. It's a good thing, because if he weren't, he might not have awakened at all. After downing some sixteen ounces of the rum, his blood alcohol level would have been more than .38 percent. The reason he felt okay initially was that it takes time for the alcohol to build up in the bloodstream. It continued to be absorbed, and when the level became high enough, his body just shut down.

"I was embarrassed, very embarrassed," said Tom. "After that everybody started calling me the Captain." He apologized to his date's parents. "Her mother was upset, but I think she felt better when I told her I knew I shouldn't have done that." Still, Tom had little concern about the risk he took and, indeed, neither did his date's father, who treated it strictly as boys-will-be-boys type stuff. "He thought it was the funniest thing in the world," said Tom.

## Beyond the Fun and Games

Other none-too-pleasant things can happen when you're drunk, too. Blackouts are one. This is when you forget what you did for a period of time, even if you never actually lose consciousness.

"I've blacked out before," said Allison. "It's kind of scary. I woke up the next morning and didn't know where I'd been or how I got home. Sometimes you're sitting there in biology class and all of a sudden it hits you, and you think, 'Oh yeah, now I remember.' But you don't know if it's a dream or if it really happened."

"I've had times where I don't remember where I put anything," said Lisa. "I'd wake up and couldn't find my clothes or my shoes. My money. Where's my money? Did somebody steal it? It's weird."

Donna spoke of a time she got drunk and started crying and screaming four-letter words and crashing into things. She blacked out through almost all of it. "I fell down the stairs and didn't even remember that. When I found out, it just scared me."

When alcohol flows, fists often are not far behind, either. Ellen said one whole side of her family is made up of very big men who are very big boozers. "Practically every time there's a family party they end up fighting with each other," she said.

"Yeah, fights get pretty wild," said Lisa. "The guys really go at it sometimes." Evan talked about times when getting drunk and having fights became almost as routine as talking. "I wouldn't care when I was drunk," he said. "I'd go after guys who were much bigger."

Vandalism is standard fare, too. Darrin's idea of a good time used to be tying one on and going out for a ride on residential streets, bashing down one mailbox after another with a baseball bat. Once, Harry felt like going for a ride and didn't have his father's car. So he hot-wired somebody else's, went out riding for a few hours, and brought it back.

## Ready or Not

And then there's another kind of adventure, or misadventure, as the case may be. The sexual kind. Many people agreed that because it lowers your inhibitions, alcohol makes it easier to relate to the opposite sex. But they did not agree with something else you hear quite a bit: that alcohol is a great aphrodisiac, that it increases desire and makes you a better partner.

Since alcohol depresses the senses, the reality is that your body is less responsive to all stimuli, the sexual variety included. "You're a lot bolder when you drink," said Tom. "Guys are more forward and girls are easier. But when it comes right down to it, it's not good to drink if you're going to have sex. You can't control your body as well. It's not as much fun. You just can't perform the same way."

And there's also the matter of getting so uninhibited that you get involved sexually when you don't really want to—or when neither party has taken the necessary precautions. The results range from regret to pregnancy.

Randi has been pregnant twice as a direct result of being drunk and not being careful. "And I have a friend, I think she's been pregnant five times by now. She was drinking and she didn't really think about anything."

Jane also regretted her sexual encounter—the one she lost a friend over. "I don't think the alcohol made me do it," she said. "But if I had been straight, I would have asked myself, 'Well, what about her, your girlfriend?' Later I regretted it, because we used to be friends and now she hates me."

## Thinking It Through

Some of those we spoke to weren't fazed by these consequences of getting drunk. Like Jane, their attitude was largely that it's just the price for having a good time. Much of it seems to stem from the belief we talked of at the very outset—that alcohol is everywhere, so really, how could it be so bad? As Karl said, "Alcohol just isn't taken that seriously." As a result, things that can happen to you when you're drinking aren't taken very seriously, either.

But this isn't the case with everyone. Many others were alarmed by the things that happened when they were drunk and vowed not to let them happen again. Others, like Tracy, are alarmed by what they see around them. Tracy has an alcoholic father whose personality changes dramatically when he's drinking. Between that and watching her friends get drunk at parties, she has observed enough to know that getting drunk is not for her.

"It changes your mind," said Tracy. "Like with my father, it makes this stuff come out of him. He can be a jerk. He argues. Normally he's not a jerk. Alcohol doesn't make you have a clear, complete mind. Someone asks you something one night, and asks again the next night, you'll probably give them two different answers.

"At parties, people will come up and say, 'Why don't you have a beer or something? How come you're not drinking?' And my feeling is that when you drink, you get your way into situations you don't want to get into. They keep asking me, and I'm thinking, 'I don't want to drink because I don't want to ruin my life the way the rest of you are.' "

Tracy is fifteen. She has tried alcohol at a wedding but is in no hurry to try it again. Sure, she sees people having fun drinking. But she also sees the fights and accidents and tears and troubles with parents. It's really pretty simple why she feels as she does about drunkenness. "You just have much more of a risk of dying while you're drinking than you do when you're not," she said.

Richard is another who takes the consequences of drunkenness seriously. "You look at people drinking too much, and you see it just makes for lots of problems. Look at the movies; you always see trouble starting in the bar. People don't know what they're doing when they're drunk. They make a lot of trouble. It makes fights. It makes people unhappy."

Richard says his father has talked to him a lot about drinking and what it can do. The message has been absorbed. "It can do a lot of damage," Richard said. "A lot of kids don't see that. At school, when they talk about alcohol, all they talk about is the good. They say, 'Oh, it makes me feel so good.' But they don't understand it fully. You don't hear them talking about getting in accidents or getting somebody pregnant, or about how it can make you want to take drugs. There are so many things in the world to appreciate. If they hadn't made alcohol, I think this world would have been a lot better off."

## Weighing Things

We've heard from both sides. From some people who look at getting drunk as the ultimate good time, and from others who feel the only thing getting drunk is good for is wreaking havoc in your life. There even have been some who have experienced both, and on the very same night; who, for a few hours, had rollicking fun, but who kept at it and overdid it and came away saying, "I'm never going to drink that way again."

The message received from those who drink seems to be that yes, you can have fun when you're drunk, but also that, yes, it's very easy to go too far and have the fun go away.

The line between a happy glow and a messy, risky disorientation is not all that clear. Because it is broken down so slowly, alcohol keeps creeping up on you, keeps spilling into your bloodstream, and affects you much more than you might have suspected. As Tracy said, "If you're going to drink, I think you need to do it slowly. Be reasonable about it. That way you'll just get relaxed, maybe a little buzzed."

A few other things about getting drunk are worth heeding. One is that the more you drink and the earlier you start, the greater your chance of becoming an alcoholic. This isn't the stuff of idle warnings; it is a statistical fact. You have a lot of things going on inside when you're a teenager. There are vast physical changes, and vast emotional ones, too. There's a natural assertion of independence, a pulling away from parents. It's a full agenda, no question.

Alcohol is a powerful drug for everybody. But with all the change and growth going on, teenagers are extra vulnerable to its mood-altering, mind-altering effects—which is precisely why many respected authorities on the subject feel very strongly that drinking shouldn't be part of the teenage social scene at all. Not until the legal age arrives, at the very least.

Evan started drinking early. He was getting drunk regularly at age eleven. He has stopped now (more from him later on this) and has learned a thing or two in his trials with booze. "Kids start way too early," he said. "It's a problem, because they can get addicted to it, like I did. And the younger they are, the worse it is. They say the less you weigh, the drunker you get. And the drunker you get, the greater the risk you'll die. To me, that's the whole thing right there: Alcohol can kill you.

"I have a lot of friends who started drinking before me and who are still at it," Evan continued. "Some of them have really serious drinking problems. Half of them are always getting kicked out of their houses or running away. Others drink for other reasons, to escape their problems, whatever. But they're heading for trouble and I fear for them."

## Chugging into Trouble

The other thing to remember is that how—and why—you drink can put you at risk, too. As we've seen, chugging hard liquor is right up there with the worst things you can do to your body. It amounts to poisoning yourself by pouring a toxic amount of a drug inside you. It makes the blood alcohol level soar and the central nervous system crawl. If you chug with any significant amount of alcohol already in you, you stand a pretty good chance of dying.

These things are not usually in the forefront of the mind of someone who's about to down a large amount of something or other. Again, we get back to alcohol being taken lightly and drinking being, for some, a big game. Even Maggie, who's not a heavy drinker at all, got caught up in the gamesmanship; you'll recall she wanted to "shock" a few friends by accepting a dare to chug a pint of brandy. This is the same person who said, "I've never been drunk. I don't want to be. I can see what it does, what happens to other people, and I don't want to go through that." And here she was putting away a pint. In one shot. Even when you're alert to the perils of alcohol abuse, it can be dangerously easy to underestimate how powerful the stuff really is.

## Why Do You Do It?

Perhaps the people most in danger of underestimating alcohol are those who need it the most. These are the people who drink—and get drunk—for a very pointed reason: to get away from their problems.

You might be thinking, "What's the difference if I drink because there's a big party, or because I want to forget about my parents' screaming at each other? Alcohol is alcohol, isn't it?"

Alcohol *is* alcohol, but why you drink makes a world of difference nonetheless. And the reason is that the more alcohol is used to escape, the greater the chance of becoming hooked on that escape. Dr. O'Brien calls drinking this way self-medication, in the sense that you're using alcohol to wash away depression, anxiety, and so on. To medicate your pain.

"It's a major problem," he said. "Drinking this way only adds to the depression and makes the situation worse. You can't cope as well and the problem only grows. That drinking helps is an absolute myth."

Ernie agrees. "I've tried that. I've used alcohol to drown my sorrows. I've gotten so mad at a person I said I would just get drunk to forget about that person for a little while. But then you get drunk and in a depressed state and it hurts five times as bad. I can't see why people do that. But they do. That's why some people are in so much trouble with their drinking."

## Resisting the Quick Fix

Problems are not always evenly distributed. Some of us have heavier loads than others at certain times in our lives. When things are feeling overwhelming, it's tempting to want to get out from under them for a while. A friend may come up to you and say, "Let's go to so-and-so's party. We'll have a few. You'll feel better." You go, you do have a few. Maybe you do feel better, for a time.

That's okay, to feel better, but the danger is that the more alcohol is used to handle things, the less able we are to handle things without it. Drinking to escape troubles is like slapping a coat of paint on a rotten board. The board will look better. But underneath, the rotting is still going on. You haven't dealt with that, just with superficialities. The board gets worse. The rot grows. And you need more and more paint to keep up. Things will only get worse until you forget the paint and deal with the board.

If you do drink, it's a good thing to ask yourself why. Try to answer as honestly as you can. If the reason is to get away from how you usually feel, to cope with a problem, to get a boost because everything seems to be screwed up, it would be an excellent idea to take a long, hard look at your drinking. It would also be an excellent idea to stop. Because the more you do this, the more used to it you get. And slowly, subtly, without you ever really knowing or sensing, you no longer just like to drink. You need to drink. And as we'll see in the next chapter, that is not a happy place to be in.

# Chapter 6

# OVER THE EDGE
## Teenage Alcoholics Tell Their Stories

He's not sure where the idea came from. He *is* sure it's wrong.

Darrin is a bright and handsome seventeen-year-old. He's talking about his misconceptions.

"I thought alcoholics were just the Skid Row bum type people" he said. "I was sure that's where they were. The real down-and-out types living by the railroad tracks."

Randi had the same idea. "I always stereotyped alcoholics. You know, there could be no doctor alcoholics. What's that? That couldn't be. That doesn't happen to those people."

Darrin and Randi found out they were wrong, and they found out the hard way. Because they're both recovering alcoholics.

We're going to hear a lot more from Darrin and Randi in this chapter, as well as from another teenage alcoholics. We'll look at how their drinking got out of hand, how they dealt with the problem (and didn't deal with it), and what finally got them on the road to recovery. They debunk quite a few myths and stereotypes along the way.

## The Box Mentality

Stereotypes are everywhere. If you think about it, you can probably come up with a dozen in a minute: House-wives aren't as smart as women who work outside the home. Italian people are involved with the Mafia. Athletes are dumb. Irish people drink a lot. Lawyers are shifty.

The list is endless. And teenagers are on it, too. Chances are you and your friends have, at some point, been unfairly lumped together by people who think: Teenagers drive too fast. They have awful taste in music. They rebel against their parents. They're reckless.

Once, as a kid, I went into a store to buy a card. I instantly sensed the storeowner's eyes upon me. I had browsed over maybe six cards when he approached. Briskly.

"You're getting the cards all musty-dusty," he said. His tone was testy, his stereotype unmistakable: All kids are a pain, and they're all on the earth to mess up my store, or possibly shoplift. I never bought one of his musty-dusty cards again.

It's wrong, and lazy, to reduce life to a bunch of boxes and labels. It's also dangerous, as Darrin and Randi discovered. Like millions of people in this society, they deluded themselves into thinking that respectable people don't become alcoholics. The flip side of this is clear: "It happens to other people. It could never happen to me."

Alcoholism has killed millions of people over the years. And the vast majority of them went to their graves thinking, "Me, an alcoholic? No way, not me." This is why alcoholism is called a disease of denial. One alcoholic put it this way: "This disease is baffling. It's insidious. It's the only disease that constantly tells you you don't have the disease."

## An Equal-Opportunity Affliction

So anyone can become an alcoholic. You can develop a problem when you're fourteen or forty, or seventy-three for that matter. You can be black or white or purple. You can be a brain surgeon, schoolteacher, or street sweeper. It can, and does, hit anybody.

We've used the term "disease" in talking about alcoholism. What does this mean? It means that a lack of willpower or a shortage of high morals has nothing to do with it. It means that the alcoholic becomes powerless over his* drinking. Alcoholics are, in the truest sense of the word, sick people. Their sickness is marked by a compulsion to drink alcohol, even as the drinking is creating problems in their lives. In most instances, they know they should stop, know the pain and hardship their drinking is causing. But they can't stop because they are addicted. They need alcohol. They crave it. This is their disease.

How you get to be an alcoholic has been a question,

---

* Here and elsewhere in this book, the male pronoun is used to refer to the alcoholic. This is only for the sake of simplicity. Females can develop drinking problems just as easily, and everything related should be considered to apply to both genders.

studied by thousands, for decades. We have very solid clues, and we know who is at risk for the disease, but still cannot pinpoint who will develop a problem and who won't. Two guys can sit on adjacent barstools and drink the same stuff in the same quantity for the same amount of time—and one can become an alcoholic while the other may not.

As we've noted earlier, the disease very definitely runs in families; if you grow up in an alcoholic home, you're four times as likely to develop a drinking problem yourself. Studies have also shown that the younger you begin to drink, the greater the chance of becoming an alcoholic.

Some problem drinkers* will tell you they were alcoholics from the very first drink. They speak of marked personality changes, of feeling a powerful urge to keep drinking, of a dramatic and soothing transformation in the way they saw the world. More common, however, is for the disease to develop gradually. Some people can drink for years before developing a problem, as was the case with Martha. She was a very moderate social drinker who liked the relaxing, mellowing effect of alcohol. She drank for twenty years, showing no indication of any problem whatsoever, before the disease took root in her. And then, seemingly out of nowhere, it hit. There were family problems and an unraveling marriage, and alcohol helped take the edge off life's burdens. She turned to it more and more. She became dependent. And then she became addicted.

This is a common pattern. The yearning for alcohol gets stronger. Much stronger. What used to be a simple feeling of wanting to drink becomes a feeling of needing

---

* The terms "problem drinker" and "alcoholic" are used interchangeably throughout the text.

to drink. Life seems unmanageable without it. The need intensifies. Alcohol becomes a crutch—and the alcoholic becomes psychologically hooked on it. The crutch eventually becomes a full-blown craving, and then physiological changes occur that make the alcoholic physically addicted. He cannot live without the stuff. It takes center stage in his life. Alcohol governs all else.

What sets this diseased progression in motion is difficult to say. Some research shows an actual genetic predisposition to alcoholism, meaning that problem drinkers have an innate inability to handle alcohol—a trait passed on from their parents, right along with their blue eyes and blond hair. Others believe the disease is more behavioral in origin—that problem drinkers, who often have great amounts of insecurity and self-doubt, learn that drinking is the easiest way to deal with their troubling feelings. They drink, they feel better. They like feeling better, they drink more.

There are no guarantees about who will and who won't become an alcoholic. But it's almost guaranteed that if you use alcohol as an escape, to handle problems and ease tensions, the disease of alcoholism will find you sooner or later. Probably sooner.

## The Road to Trouble

Darrin was ten years old, a fifth-grader, when he snuck his first drink with a thirteen-year-old friend. The day is still vivid in his memory: "We were in my friend's grandfather's garage. There was a refrigerator with all this beer. We started drinking those little pony beers, and drank a whole lot of them. I didn't like the taste, but I saw everybody else doing it and they seemed to like it, so I thought I would do it. We did it again the next week.

When my friend's grandfather died, we starting drinking other stuff, hard stuff, they had in there, too. Pretty soon we had the run of the place; we'd just go in and shut the garage door and start drinking. I started regularly getting drunk on weekends. I liked it. I don't know why. I felt like it gave me more energy. It made me feel better than I felt normally. For that five or six or ten hours, I didn't think about what was bothering me."

What bothered his parents was when Darrin started coming home reeking of booze. "My mother couldn't believe it," Darrin said. "You don't see that many ten-year-olds getting drunk." There would be regular family battles over his drinking. "My mother was always trying to get me to stop, so I would not drink for a couple of weeks, just to prove to her that I could control it." Darrin thought this was proof he wasn't an alcoholic. Another misconception.

## Fooling Himself

Many people think you have to drink all day, every day, to be a problem drinker. Or that you have to drink as soon as you get up in the morning. As a result, they think if they stop for a period of time—a day, a week, even a month—that it's proof they don't have a problem with it. As Darrin says, "I knew, or thought I knew, I wasn't an alcoholic because I never drank during the week."

This simply isn't true. Even if the alcoholic doesn't drink for a period of time, the underlying disease is still there. Which means that the alcoholic will go back to the bottle at some point, and when he does, the drinking will fire right back up, very quickly. One of the things that makes alcoholism so wicked is that it's a progressive disease. You don't just get the craving and then become fond of drinking too much. It would be far easier to cope with—and far less lethal—if this were the case. What happens is that the compulsion becomes progressively worse. The drinking interferes more and more with day-to-day living. Life becomes a steady, downward spiral—a spiral ruled by getting alcohol inside you.

Darrin's mother tried everything to get him to stop. She even tried bribing him. She bought him a motorcycle, with the stipulation that he could only drive it when he was sober. But for all her good intentions, Darrin's mother, at that point, was treating it as though he were simply choosing to drink too much, that he was a lush with no willpower and he darn well better stop. She had a hard time accepting that it wasn't that Darrin didn't want to control his drinking, it was that he couldn't. No bribe or threat was going to cure his disease, any more than it would cure cancer.

## A Life Falls Apart

Before long, alcohol seriously disrupted Darrin's life. By the time he was fourteen, his drinking had almost killed him several times. There were trips to the emergency room, run-ins with the police, and dozens of episodes where he couldn't remember what he had done while he was drunk. One time Darrin drove four hundred miles after drinking several six-packs of beer. He got into an accident and to this day doesn't know where he drove or how the accident occurred.

Darrin knew, deep down, he had a problem. A serious one. He was just terrified to face it. "I would've sworn at you if you had said to me I had a problem," said Darrin.

"I knew, but I still wanted to do it. I didn't want help yet. I liked being how I was, in a way. It's hard to explain. I didn't like waking up the next day and not remembering anything and finding out what I'd done, driving around, getting in fights. Once I almost got strangled to death. I was talking to this guy's girlfriend, just talking, except I didn't know she was with somebody. Next thing I knew there was a rope around my neck. I didn't like hearing about all that stuff, but I did like the feeling. It just made me feel better. I got away from everything for that time."

## The Power of Denial

Darrin's attitude is right out of the alcoholic textbook. Denial is a strange thing. It would seem nearly impossible to deny something when it's such a problem. But alcoholics are great at it, and for a very clear reason: fear.

When we're really afraid of something, there's a great human urge to run from it. Ignoring it, downplaying it, is a lot easier than taking it on. When I was a teenager, I had a pretty bad skin problem for a time. I did not want to deal with it or think about it. I did not want to go to a dermatologist to take care of it. So I didn't. I just stuffed it. Ignored it completely. I walked around as if I had baby-smooth skin. Classic denial.

I eventually came around. The condition worsened and there was no more pretending it wasn't a problem. I went to the doctor, cared for it, and things turned out okay. But there's no underestimating the power of the human mind to turn away from unpleasant—and frightening—things.

With problem drinkers, first they deny that they could

ever have a problem with alcohol. Later, they deny the seriousness of the problem once it has begun. They have no control over their drinking, they're terrified, they deny.

## From Bad to Worse

Darrin's need to escape got more and more urgent. His disease progressed. Darrin was in big trouble. Nine times, he was in detox units (hospital wards where people dry out) or rehabilitation centers. Once when he was drinking, he fell off a dam and plummeted fifty-five feet into water. Miraculously, he was unhurt. He got into dealing drugs to get drinking money. His parents were ready to throw him out of the house. The cops were constantly on his tail. Darrin was sixteen years old and, by his own account, a maniac. "I was crazy when I drank," he said. "I did insane things." You look at him and listen to him, so soft-spoken and clear-headed, and you can hardly believe it as he tells of carrying guns, dealing drugs, attempting suicide, getting in wicked fights, and more. You realize he was totally enslaved by his addiction.

"I thought I drank to get away from my problems," he said. "What I finally had to face was that the drinking was actually *causing* the problems."

He fooled himself for a long time with that I-only-drink-on-weekends bit. Finally, he could fool himself no more. Finally, his once-fierce denial got shattered. It took a powerful, painful experience to do it. This is sometimes called hitting rock bottom—getting so low and in so much distress that you simply can't deny any longer.

Darrin's bottom, and his last drink, came at a party, when somebody slipped something into his beer, sending him on a nightmarish trip that lasted nearly two weeks.

"When I woke up, I was in a psychiatric hospital. My head was in a straightjacket," he recalled. "I couldn't see my feet. I thought the walls were moving. I was crazy. Sometimes I would have spells where I was totally off the wall. Then I would be normal again. I didn't think it was ever going to stop. It was awful. That's when I finally knew I had to get help."

## Getting Sober, Staying Sober

He went to another rehab center, but this time was different, because he truly wanted help. Recovering from alcoholism is an extremely difficult process. It is not just deciding to stop drinking. It is about dealing, first, with physical withdrawal, which can be hellish all by itself. And it is about changing an entire lifestyle, your behavioral patterns, your thought processes, attitudes, your whole way of looking at the world. It is facing life, for the first time in years (usually), without the escape hatch of booze, without using alcohol to relieve your pain, soothe your worries, make everything right. It's also hard because recovery calls for staying away from alcohol permanently. You don't just dry out and then go back, trying to be more careful. The disease is still there; if you go back to drinking, it picks up where it left off. Alcoholism doesn't get cured; it just gets controlled—by the drinker coming to grips with the compulsion, realizing he needs to change his way of life, and by staying sober.

Today Darrin's life has completely turned around. He has a promising future in his trade. He has a busy social life, much of it centered around friends he has met through Alcoholics Anonymous, a support group that has meetings in thousands of communities across the country, and indeed, across the world. He has even started two youth A.A. groups, helping his own sobriety while at the same time helping others recover from their problem with alcohol.

"It's phenomenal now," said Darrin. "The difference is unbelievable. I have so much more energy. I go biking ten miles every morning. I do things that are good for me. I used to be so sick. Sick physically, and sick in the head.

"But maybe the biggest difference is with my mother. I can go out and come home late and she won't worry. I can stay over at a friend's house and she won't think I'm lying. Used to be she would ask me questions for a half hour over something like that. She really can trust me now.

"I feel like I know so much more now," Darrin continued. "About myself, and about other people. All I used to know about was going out with my friends and partying. I feel like I'm accepted for being myself now, for who I am, not for how much I can drink. I have what I want. I feel like I can deal with whatever problems come up." Darrin smiled. And then he said, "I like myself a lot better now."

## Running Away

Her skin is smooth and her face is pretty. Her blue eyes are clear and radiant. They weren't always that way. Randi is sixteen. She has been through hell with alcohol.

"Most teenagers think you can't become an alcoholic so young," said Randi. "They think you have to be drinking for thirty years and be forty years old, and that because you may not drink every day, you can't have a problem." Randi offers herself as proof of yet another misconception.

Randi's first drinking experience was at a family Christmas party when she was nine. Her alcoholic uncle kept feeding her rum and Cokes. He thought it was funny to see his little niece stumble around, lose control of herself, not be able to speak clearly.

Randi got drunk, passed out, blacked out, and got sick her very first time. She drank very infrequently after that, until age thirteen. Life at home had become unbearable. She had endured years of sexual and physical abuse by her stepfather. A cauldron of anger and guilt and helplessness had been building inside her, and it finally burst. "I just flew off the handle," she said. She was filled with hurt and despair. She discovered that alcohol was very good at numbing these feelings.

"I didn't think there was anything wrong with using alcohol this way," she said. "It made me forget anything going on, any problem, it just made me forget. It helped me escape my feelings. I was always very lonely and depressed, and I always thought drinking would make it better." The feelings would get soothed, temporarily. "But things never got better, only worse," she said.

Randi started hanging out with juniors and seniors— the "alcohol crowd," as she calls it. "To go out on a Friday night, there needed to be alcohol in the car or it just wasn't worth going out," she said.

She had always been a fine student, but by freshman year, Randi was absent 113 out of the 181 school days. "My grades went completely down the tubes. But, of course, I didn't have a problem. Not me." Randi laughed at her sarcasm.

More and more, drinking just seemed to be the thing

to do. She drank not only to forget, but to have fun, to be cool. "I think I always saw the glamor involved with alcohol. The adults sitting around drinking a glass of wine or whatever. I put it together with the social scene." She could not imagine life without it.

Randi's progression was rapid. She advanced from Friday night parties to weekend-long alcohol binges. "I needed it so much toward the end, it was such a desperation for it, that I would drink before I went to school . . . if I went to school."

She was committed to a psychiatric hospital for a year because of several drunken suicide attempts. She lied about her drinking. She carved a hole in the floor of her room to hide bottles. Still, she had denial.

"I didn't want to blame my problems on my drinking," she said. "I was addicted to alcohol, but I just thought I was tired, or getting sick. I never really put my problems together with my drinking until later."

## False Impressions

Part of the problem was Randi's taking alcohol lightly. Like so many of us, she saw how pervasive alcohol was and assumed it had to be pretty harmless. She saw it flowing in bars and restaurants, and how it was the focal point of just about every weekend activity in her crowd. She saw beautiful people drinking it on television, having fun, being carefree, living the good life. She did not see—nor will she, or any of us, ever see—one of these beautiful people having a problem with their drinking. Or having a car accident, or getting in a fight, or even just getting depressed from alcohol.

Said Randi, "People knew that with a drug like cocaine you can become addicted to it quickly. That's very clear to them. But they don't think you can become addicted to alcohol, except after years and years of drinking. I think teenagers get that message from their parents. Parents say it's okay to drink but just don't do drugs. They don't link the two together." The double message strikes again.

"People are pretty naive about alcohol," Randi said. "They don't know what it can do to them. Sometimes I think it will take for somebody to die from it before they know what's really going on."

Like Darrin, Randi also had to go through living hell before she finally quit. "I did things that normal people just don't do," she said. "I would lie down in the middle of a main street, stupid things like that. I stole a lot, from my parents and grandparents and friends, and I definitely wasn't brought up to do that." She slept around a lot, too. "I got a pretty bad reputation," she said. She also got pregnant twice, and had one abortion and one miscarriage. "I regret that most of all," she said.

## On the Brink

She was in and out of institutions. There were repeated suicide attempts. At one point, she was put on Antabuse, a drug that makes you violently sick if combined with alcohol. "I drank when I was on it," Randi said. "It was insane. I was deathly ill." Day after day, she would promise herself she would not drink. "And by the end of the day, I would be drunk."

It all got to be too much. The denial finally began to crumble. She began to see alcohol wasn't the solution, but the cause of the chaos her life had dissolved into. Meanwhile, a close friend had made a similar realization and had started going to Alcoholics Anonymous. "I'd partied with him a lot," she said. "I figured, 'If he has a problem, maybe I do, too.' " Randi went to an A.A. meeting.

"I heard people talking about their experiences and feelings, and it was like they were talking about me. They were telling my life story. I just pretty much gave into it at that point. I couldn't control my drinking."

She also took a simple, twenty-question test someone had given her to determine if she had a drinking problem. "I was honest on it. I did come out as having a problem. Finally, I said, 'That's enough. I'm quitting. I'm sick of it.' "

## Starting Over

Randi had been in A.A. for eight months when we talked. "Sometimes it's hard, very hard," she said, "because I'm still in high school and there's a lot of drinking around. When I have a problem in my life, it becomes harder. But then I just think back and remember what alcohol did to me. I know I have this disease, and that if I went back to drinking, I could die from it." As they teach in A.A., Randi works at staying sober one day at a time. She tries not to project about how hard it will be to be sober for the rest of her life, and tries to avoid getting too burdened by past regrets or future worries. She seeks to put all that she can into each day. Most important of all, she seeks to stay away from drinking.

Life has begun anew. "I have real friends now," she said. "I have people I know and can trust. My drinking friends, we just got wasted and used each other. Now, when any problem comes up, I can get it out. People will listen to me. I can talk about things, and I've dealt with some of the back issues from my childhood. My self-

esteem is up a little. I don't feel super-great about myself, but I feel like I'm okay today, and that's a big step,
because I always thought I was garbage. I don't need
alcohol to feel good. And that's something I never thought
would happen.

"I wouldn't give up being sober for anything in the
world," Randi said. "It's the best thing that ever happened to me. It's amazing, with everything that happened to me. All I can say is that what I have now is a
gift from God."

## Of Fights—and Flight

For Evan, right from the beginning, the escape was the
thing. His parents were going through a tough time.
Their fights were becoming more and more frequent.
Evan wanted to get away, so he headed for the bowling
alley, where a bunch of his friends had taken to hanging
out. He also headed for alcohol.

"I drink to escape the tension at home," he said. "I
went out and got drunk the first night they had a really
bad fight, and it got so I was looking forward to every
weekend, so I could get drunk again." And that's just
about what Evan did, from age eleven to age thirteen.

Many of the kids in the group were older, and all were
heavily into partying. Evan went along. "I probably passed
out ten times in those two years," he said. He would get
drunk and stay drunk for two or three or four days at a
shot. Occasionally he would drink before school, but
even when he didn't, there were constant run-ins with
teachers, and lots of other people, too. Fights were a
regular event at the bowling alley. One night he saw a
friend get stabbed. Another night, he and a friend were

walking home, drunk, when suddenly a car pulled over. The driver got out. And pulled out a gun.

Evan had studied karate for two years. It came in handy as he executed a spinning kick that sent the gun flying. He and his friend pummeled the guy briefly, then ran as fast as their drunken bodies would taken them. It wasn't fast, but fast enough. Another time when he was drunk, Evan stole someone's pocketbook and took money to buy booze. Sometimes he would go out and randomly slash tires. "I would never do anything like that without drinking," he said. He hung out a lot and drank a lot. His sister confronted him, tried to get him to quit. "I said, 'I'll quit, I'll quit,' but I kept drinking." He was very close to getting in very big trouble. One day, it all hit him.

"I saw my friends and all the stupid things we were getting into, and I just didn't want to be a part of it anymore. I didn't want to get in fights. I didn't want to get killed." Evan came to a realization. "I'm an alcoholic," he said. For whatever reason—these things aren't precise—his denial wasn't so formidable as Darrin's or Randi's. He accepted the mess alcohol was making of life comparatively quickly. It spared him a whole lot more messes.

"I just saw that alcohol wasn't the answer," said Evan. "I realized what I was doing was wrong. I realized you're not supposed to use alcohol to get out your feelings or to escape. The best thing to do is to talk to an adult. I mean, alcohol isn't the answer to anything. The problems didn't go away." The more he looked at his friends, the more he saw this was true. "They were acting so weird. I didn't like it. I didn't want to end up like that, too," he said.

## Heart-to-Heart

Evan approached his father. "I was shaking, I was so nervous about it." But he felt strongly that he needed to talk about his problem, get his father's advice and, he hoped, his support.

"I'm concerned about my drinking," Evan began. He explained what he'd been doing and why he was concerned—almost all of it a shock to his father—and they went on to have a great talk about it. "I think one of the best things you can do is go to your parent, if he will really understand what you're going through," Evan said. Evan promised his father he wouldn't drink anymore. So far he has stuck to it.

"I realized it was very hard to quit, because I was addicted to it," he said. "A lot of people say alcohol isn't addictive. Well, it is. People depend on it. I craved it a lot, especially when I was in school, getting into trouble with the teachers and all that." A lot of people also say that beer and wine, particularly, can be consumed without worry about getting hooked. This misconception states: "You can only really have a problem with hard liquor." But as Evan and many, many others have discovered, you can become an alcoholic on beer or wine or any other variety of alcohol. Name your drink of choice— fruit-flavored brandy, wine coolers, Cold Duck—and you can get addicted to it. Beneath the flavor and color and the other stuff they throw in, it's the same substance: ethyl alcohol.

"Everywhere you look it seems like there's somebody with alcohol in their hands," said Evan. "The way I see it, I got off easy. I stopped drinking before everything got really bad. If I had kept drinking, what would have happened could have changed my whole life. I'd probably be in juvenile court or something because of some-thing I did when I was under the influence of alcohol. I was bad, and it was getting worse."

Evan has worked at filling his life with other, more healthful activities. He's picked up new hobbies and gotten serious about playing guitar in a band. "They're all people who had abused alcohol," Evan said. They all saw the problems it was making. And they all decided their lives would be much the better without it.

## Troubling Trends

"There are a lot of teenagers out there in trouble," said Evan. "I mean, if a kid like me can get into it at eleven, then there have got to be many older teenagers who are a lot worse than I am."

Randi agreed. "There's a big drug problem in my school, but I think alcohol is the biggest problem of all. The highlight of every weekend is the keg parties Friday and Saturday nights. Wherever you go, it's like, 'Let's bring some alcohol.' Everything revolves around it. People just don't think it can do anything to them."

Evan knows how easy it would be to slip back into drinking. But like Randi and Darrin, he has developed tremendous respect for what alcohol can do—and what it *did* do to him. "I pray to God it doesn't happen," he said.

He also prays that he doesn't let that misconception steer him wrong again. The one that got him started, the one that makes problem drinking so difficult: the it-could-never-happen-to-me syndrome.

"That's exactly what I thought," he said. "I'm the only one in my family that doesn't smoke. I always said, I'm not that dumb, I'm not going to smoke. I tried it, and then quit. I figured it would be the same with alcohol. Then I started drinking and getting into trouble. A couple of times along the line, I said, 'Maybe I have a little drinking problem.' But then I would come right back and say, 'No, that won't happen to me. I won't let it.'

"It's so strange," said Evan. "Because so many people say that, and then it turns around and happens to them. I didn't believe it could happen, but it did."

## Spreading the Word

Darrin thinks getting that message across to younger kids is the best way to start getting this disease under control. "I want to tell them how dangerous it is," he said. "Tell them what can happen. I tell them what happened to me, and let them know, yes, it could happen to you. You never know. Maybe you'll drink and never have a problem. Or maybe you'll drink and by the time you're thirty years old you'll be living down at the railroad tracks. Most won't be. Most won't get to that point. But you never know.

"It's not worth drinking," Darrin said. "All it does is mess up your thoughts and the way you act. It doesn't really do anything for you. People who are retarded, they'd probably give up the rest of their lives to have one day to be like we are, to be normal. And we have a whole life of being normal, and we go out and get messed up—and act retarded.

"It's not worth the risk," said Darrin. "Not even worth getting started on it." He talked some more about how easy it is to get into it, about how so many kids drink instead of trying to deal with their problems. And then he talked again about his new life. His rich, sober life.

Darrin said, "I get up every day and say a prayer that

I'm not going to drink for today. And every night, I say a prayer, and thank God that I was able to do it. I do that every day. I'd like to be able to do that forever."

He never thought it could happen, but it did. And now Darrin, along with Randi and Evan, has struggled and fought and rebuilt his life.

They all still have the disease, because it doesn't leave. But they're all recovering from it. They've done it with a lot of work and a lot of courage, the kind it takes to admit, "I'm in trouble. I can't control myself. I need help." They've been through hell, but they've made it back, and that makes them very special.

"Life has never been better," said Darrin.

# Chapter 7

# DRINKING AND DRIVING
## A Sure Road to Disaster

Maggie was leaving the party. She needed a ride and a friend offered to take her. Maggie decided to accept. It was a bad decision.

"He seemed fine," said Maggie. They got in the car and he started driving. Which was when Maggie found out he wasn't so fine after all. "He was drunk," she said.

Maggie is a smart and perceptive eighteen-year-old. She prides herself on being sensible and responsible, and the fact is, she was pretty sensible that night. The friend she drove to the party with was clearly bombed. Maggie wasn't about to go with him, or let him go anywhere, so she took his car keys and left them with the party host. Then she made other arrangements to get home—and made her mistake.

"I didn't realize he was drunk until I was already halfway home," she said. "We were on this curvy road and he was barely on the road half the time. It was one of the scariest things I've ever been through. We had to tell him, 'No, you need to be over here more, no, not that far, now a little over here.' " It was two-thirty in the morning and few other cars were around, so her big fear was not so much hitting another car. It was slamming into a telephone pole or some other object.

"I will never get in the car again with someone who had just been drinking," she said.

## Another Chance

Maggie is very fortunate. For her, there will be other rides, other decisions to make. Others who have made the same miscalculation—tens of thousands of others— never made it home.

Awareness of the perils of drinking and driving has never been greater. Every young person we talked to confirmed this. Over and over, the message was the same: "You hear much more about it now. You see movies. You get pamphlets. There are commercials on TV. A lot more kids have a 'designated driver' if they're going out and they expect to drink. The warnings are all over the place."

Thanks to the efforts of such programs as Students Against Driving Drunk (SADD), Mothers Against Drunk Drivers (MADD), Safe Rides, and RID (Remove Intoxicated Drivers), as well as those of corporations and state and local agencies, the entire country has gotten a crash course—pun intended—on this awful problem.

That's the positive news. Not so positive is that the problem is still enormous. It's better, but a long, long way from being eliminated. We said it earlier, but it's worth repeating: Alcohol-related accidents are the leading cause of death among teenagers. Ten thousand teen-agers die every year in such accidents. About three-quar-ters of a million people suffer serious injuries because of drunk drivers. The total cost of this drunken devastation is estimated to be $5 billion. The human cost is nothing that can be calculated.

## "Don't Worry, I'm Fine"

Alcohol is devious. It affects you, even when you're 100 percent positive that it doesn't. That's what makes it so easy to get behind the wheel, even if you've had something to drink. It's also what makes it such a menace.

Laurie talked about going to the drag races with her father and a friend of his. "His friend was totally gone. He was barely walking," she said. He drove home. He said he was fine.

Laurie said her father was less drunk, but still under the influence. "I said, 'Dad, let me drive home,' and he said, 'No, no. I'm okay. Don't worry about it!' " Laurie was certain he should not be driving. But he was "fine." She spent the trip cowering in the back seat. "I just kept saying, please, Dad, let's just make it home."

Laurie has seen the same attitude among her friends. "They'll be drinking and then they'll get in their cars. They say it will be no problem."

Ernie says that even with all the campaigns, drunken driving is common. "Kids just don't see that drinking and driving is dangerous," he said. "They think, 'Oh, we'll be fine.' They try it once when they've got a buzz and they see it's easy and then try it once more and they're a little more buzzed and before they know it they're doing it when they're outright drunk, and they crash. They don't even see it coming." Ernie and his girlfriend work out a system, depending on who's driving. "If she's driving, I can drink a little," he said. "If I'm driving, I don't touch anything."

Said Allison, "This guy was at my house once. He insisted he was okay to drive home. He couldn't even stand up. And he was saying, 'I can drive, I can drive.'"

"I was in tears. I didn't want him going like that. But I couldn't stop him, no matter what I did." The guy made it home. Allison said, "I have no idea how."

Karen doesn't drive yet; she's only fourteen. But she hasn't had a great role model in the DWI department. "Over the holidays my father drove really drunk," she said. "If my mother wasn't with him, he would've killed us all. He didn't know anything. He couldn't even walk. He was so drunk he went into our neighbors' house instead of ours. But he wanted to drive and he did." This is the same parent who Karen says forbids her to go to the movies with her friends because he's afraid of what trouble she'll get into.

Miguel has a friend who insists he's not only fine after drinking, he says he's *better*. "He drinks a lot," Miguel said, "and he always says he drives really well when he's buzzed. But I don't want to drive with him when he's drunk. I'll take the keys away from him first."

## Internal Dialogue

"It's like alcohol talks to you," said Warren. "It's saying, 'I'm not messing you up; you're in complete control.' And it says that even when you *are* messed up." He added, "Nobody drives when they're drunk thinking they're screwed up." Warren admits he has been fooled by this himself. "I've driven after drinking. Never when I was bombed, but when I definitely was over the limit.

And I know I should not have done it." He never had trouble, but says he isn't ever doing it again. The message has reached him. "I'm quitting while I'm ahead. Why be stupid about it?"

Still, it's hard. "You may be at a party and you haven't had much, you just want to get in the car," he said. "Most times, you really, truly think you're perfectly fine to drive."

And virtually every time, you're really, truly not fine. Remember what we looked at in Chapter 2: that studies show that with just .05 percent alcohol in your blood (roughly two drinks for a 150-pound person) you are twice as likely to have an accident. This is only half of the usual legal blood alcohol limit of .10 percent. Which means that well before you have trouble with the law, you can have trouble with your driving. It's also worth knowing that with .15 percent blood alcohol, your odds on having an accident are twenty-five times greater.

And they're greater for any sort of accident—even if you're not in a car. Miguel talked of riding home on his bike after doing some drinking with a friend. "I was going through downtown and I turned to the left and a car beeped at me, and the next thing I knew I had practically steered right into a parked car. I noticed my bike was going right and left, zigzagging. I said, 'Oh wow. I better not do this again.' I was scared I was going to get into an accident."

## Inner Limits, Outer Limits

How much alcohol affects you is a function of several factors, including your weight and body type (as noted earlier, the more you weigh and the more muscular you are, the more water your body contains to dilute the liquor). But virtually everybody is affected sooner than you would think. Much sooner, in fact.

For instance, using the formula from Chapter 2, we now that if you're a 125-pound female, you will very likely be legally intoxicated after, say, three five-ounce glasses of wine. You will be impaired—and shouldn't drive—even after two such drinks.

It's also important to remember that it takes the body more than an hour to fully metabolize the alcohol in one of these drinks. So if drinking is done over several hours at a faster rate than this, drunkenness will surely result.

And don't forget what we discussed earlier: The only thing that sobers you up is time. A friend of mine used to swear that if he drove with his head out the window for a short while, he would get lucid in a hurry. This may have felt nice and cleared a cobweb or two, but it did not do a thing to his blood alcohol level. Likewise, you can forget the cold showers, hot coffee, short walks, exercise sessions, vast amounts of water, and all the other alleged sobering schemes we looked at earlier. You stop drinking and you wait. That's how alcohol wears off. That's the only way.

## Dulled and Distorted

How exactly does alcohol impair you? It seeps into the brain and nervous system, and thus hinders your judgment (mental and physical). You may think you have plenty of room to pass in front of an oncoming car, when in reality you may not. Or you'll try it anyway, even if it's a little tight. Carefully weighing risks is not something people who have been drinking normally do.

Liquor also impairs your vision, your ability to judge speed, and, perhaps most importantly, your reflexes. Remember, booze slows your system down. Even a small amount can significantly decrease your reaction time. If you've spent any time at all in a car and you've ever had a close call, you know how critical every millisecond can be.

Allison recalls being in the backseat on the way home from a party. She felt a little drunk, she said. "I was watching the driver go around turns and avoid parked cars, and I just kept thinking, "If I had been driving, there's no way I would have seen that car. Or there's no way I could've made that turn. It was pretty scary."

Jerry was in the backseat once, too. He was riding with three friends, and his friends' parents were in the front. They were not far from home. "His mom asked us if we wanted to stop for ice cream," Jerry said. He would not remember anything else for a while.

"It was a two-lane road and we were going along fine, and then all of a sudden there were two headlights right in our path," said Jerry. "I didn't hear any yells. I just saw the car coming at us."

The car was going very fast, fifty or sixty in a thirty-mile-per-hour zone. The oncoming headlights bore in at them. There was a turn. The driver, who was drunk, could not make it. His car slammed head on into the car Jerry was in, rolled over the top of it, and then careened into another.

The moments following the accident were all a blur for Jerry. Bodies were strewn everywhere, alive but in shock. There was panic and screaming. The car was totaled. One of the boys took off. "He was trying to shake everybody and nobody woke up, and I think he thought everybody was dead and he got scared," said Jerry.

They were all rushed to the hospital. Jerry had a concussion and seizures, and was in the hospital for a couple of weeks. The seizures persisted, off and on, for months. He got off lightly. "My friend's father, his whole face is held together by metal plates," said Jerry. His friend, Jim, suffered a fractured skull, a shattered elbow, and months afterward was still undergoing therapy because he could not yet walk or speak properly.

"Now I hate drunk drivers," said Jerry. "I hear anything about people drinking when they drive, I just want to rip their heads off."

## Avoiding Trouble

In Jerry's case, there was really no way to avoid this horrible experience. He was in a car and it was being driven responsibly and they just got plowed into by a drunk. It's awful. But it happens.

But often you *can* do things to limit your risk. You can make choices—to drive, or not to drive, to ride along, or not ride along—that might spare you a lot of pain and trouble. And maybe, one day, your life.

It's easy to say, "I'll never drive drunk." It's not always easy to follow through on it. Obviously there's no simple, step-by-step answer here; if there were the problem wouldn't be so dreadful. But one thing you can do is make yourself constantly aware of that deviousness we looked at before; that false confidence alcohol breeds, the phony certainty that you really are fine when you definitely are not.

If you've been drinking, even if you've been drinking a little, remind yourself of this indisputable fact: You are not going to be able to drive your best, even if you are rock-solid sure you are. SO DON'T DO IT! While you're at it, you might want to tell yourself that there are morgues coast to coast that have handled bodies whose last words were, "I'll be fine." Or "I'm only going around the corner."

Maggie has a somewhat different deterrent. "It's what happened to my older sister," she said. "She was involved in a car accident after she was drinking. She wasn't out-and-out drunk, but she was above the intoxicated level and she sideswiped a car."

The authorities showed up. Maggie's sister—nice girl from a perfectly respectable family—was taken to police headquarters.

The phone rang in the middle of the night. "It was the police," said Maggie. "They said, 'Mr. Fletcher, We've got your daughter down here at headquarters on a DWI. Would you please come down and post bail?'

"Thank God, no one got hurt," said Maggie. "But still, it's on her record and she had to go through six months of courses. And that phone call . . . The whole thing just convinced me, I'm never going to drink and drive. I don't want to get stuck in that position."

## Thinking It Through

Like Maggie, a number of those interviewed said that making yourself think—and think hard—about the possible consequences is a good way to stick to a vow not to drive impaired.

Said Allison, "I would be scared to do it. And I think about that. What would I do if I had my friends in the car and I killed them? Then what would I do? How would that make me feel? And what would my parents do to me? It's pretty scary if your father has to pick you up at the police station because you were drinking and driving."

Leslie says some basic forethought has prevented her from ever driving with someone who has been drinking. "I always make sure I'm going to be with somebody who won't drink," she said. "It's like swimming, where they teach you the buddy system. I guess I learned it well. I figure if I'm going to be mature, I better act it and team up with a buddy who doesn't drink."

Martin's resolve never to drive drunk stiffened several years ago. He was working for a towing company. He got a call to go to an accident site. "I stepped on something," he said. "I looked down and it was half a motorcycle helmet, and it was full of blood. The next morning, my mother tells me that one of her best friends' daughters died in that accident."

She had left a bar on the cycle. They got on the highway. "They weren't sober, but they were in the right lane," said Martin. The oncoming car, however, was not. The impact was head-on. For the young girl and the motorcycle driver, it was over.

"Drinking and driving is screwed up," said Martin. "If drunk driving had a logo, it would be something with no boundaries. It would just be victims all over the place. There's nobody it doesn't affect.

"Drinking plus driving is a deadly weapon. As much as a loaded gun or a knife. A car is deadly enough by itself. Why add alcohol to it? I've never driven drunk. I've left my car and I've walked. I refuse to do it." There's far too much to lose, said Martin.

He talked again of the victim of the crash. "She was nineteen, beautiful, smart, going to college. She had everything going for her." And that's it. She's gone. "Her father has never been the same," Martin said. "He wants to kill the kid." The kid (the other driver) went through a rehab program and is a free man. "He's out walking the streets. Is that fair?" said Martin. "But it happens everyday. That really bothers me."

# A Preventive Pact

Another way some people insure they won't drive drunk is by making a pact with a friend. Long before it's party time, you talk openly with your friend and authorize him or her to forbid you to drive if you have anything to drink. You make up specific guidelines (say, two drinks or more and driving is out). You make them clear. And you speak to your friend beforehand, so when it comes time to go and the liquor is telling you, "You're fine, let's get going," you're friend will remind you of the vow.

By going public with it in this way, some people are better able to face the facts and quiet that wicked everything-will-be-swell tape. It makes you stop and think—and those are healthy processes. Potentially life-saving processes. The alcohol is telling you, "C'mon, let's go. It'll be no sweat. You'll just be extra careful. You're not going far. You're a good driver. You'll be responsible." The tape goes on and on. It's critical to know that it's giving you bad—even lethal—information.

Allison has made a deal with her friend, Weslie. "I told her that if I've had anything to drink, just don't let me drive. I don't care what I've had or what I'm saying or anything else. Don't let me do it. If I'm drunk, take my keys. Knock me out if you have to. I don't want to die and I don't want to kill anybody else. I'll probably be mad at you that night, but I'll probably thank you the next morning."

Allison has made it clear this applies even when she is just a little buzzed. "That's when I know I'll be thinking, 'Oh sure, I can do it. I'll be okay,' " she said. "That's what I'm most worried about. That's why I want a friend around to say, 'No, you can't.' "

## Getting Taken for a Ride

Making a personal and steadfast vow never to drive when you've been drinking is a very important step. But it won't do you a whole lot of good if you're not every bit as careful about who you allow to drive you.

Rita talked about how hard this can be. "Think about how many times you just say, 'I'm only going around the corner. We're not going far. Just down the road. It'll be okay.' You do that a lot. You don't really think about it. You think, 'We're going to be fine.'"

Added Allison, "You say you'll never drink and drive yourself, but then you'll get in the car with someone else who has been drinking, because it's just so easy. You don't think of it as much, for some reason."

But you need to think of it every bit as much, Allison and many others agreed. Because the harsh truth is that you can die just as easily in somebody else's car as you can in your own.

Still, saying "No thanks, I don't want to go along" can be tough.

"If someone is really drunk, you wouldn't get in the car with them," Rita said. "But if they're just a little tipsy, you think, 'Well, it's okay, they've had a couple and maybe it's not a great idea to be driving, but it's okay.' When you watch the SADD movies, you see how dangerous it is and it really hits you and it's really sad. But once you're out there, you don't think about it as much. If you have to go home and your friend who's driving is just a little buzzed, it's so easy to just go with them."

Rita has done precisely this, quite a few times. "You're in the car, and even if they look all right, it changes when they're behind the wheel. You can get really paranoid. Even if they're driving okay, you think of the movies. You get very scared." Rita knows the better option—by a large margin—is to think of the movies before you get in the car. "They're your friends and you trust them and think they're all right to drive," she said. "But they're not." So you make other travel plans. You do not ride, even with your best friend in the world, if that person has had something to drink.

## Calling Home

More than ever, the other travel plans teenagers are making involve their parents. Thanks in good part to the SADD contract (in which the parent agrees to pick up the teenager if he calls, and agrees to do so with no hassle, third degree, or lecture until the issue can be discussed the next day), this seems more and more of an option.

Said Ernie, "My parents know that I've learned when to stop. But this one time I was at a party and I wasn't really drunk or anything, but I just felt I shouldn't drive. I called them and said, 'I don't feel I should drive. If you want to come and get me that's fine, otherwise I'll just stay here for tonight.' They said, 'No problem,' and the next day they even thanked me."

Added Donald, "I think parents should talk to their child and say, 'Well, we don't want you to drink, but if you're going to drink, we'd like to know where you are and we want you to know that if you need a ride home, call us.' "

"Maybe they want to yell at you when that happens," said Ernie, "but they know you're doing something good and something smart, so they won't."

In some cases, maybe your parents *will* be upset. "They

always say, 'Call us if you need us; we won't be mad,' "
said Rita, "but then when you do they are mad. Then
they say, 'Don't go out with that friend again,' or something like that. That's why I never want to call them. I
think it's an empty gesture."

Others agreed that sometimes their parents are upset,
as Rita said, even if the parents told them to call. But
many of those interviewed said they would make the
call home regardless, if the choice came down to calling
or driving drunk. "Maybe the reaction won't be what
you'd like. Maybe you'll get the third or fourth degree,"
said Allison. "But look at what the alternative is. I'd
rather be alive and have them a little upset with me."

## Going Along?

We've looked at the pressure to go with the flow when
you're drinking. There can be pressure when it comes to
riding with a friend, too. Weslie talked about having a
few inside you, when somebody suggests everybody go
someplace. "All your friends are going and you want to
go, too," she said. "That's where the peer pressure comes
in. You really want to go and you're really not buzzed at
all, and because everybody wants to go, they're all saying,
'Oh, it will be no problem.' But you just have to put the
pressure aside. You can't care what anyone thinks. It's
your life. You just have to come straight out and tell
them, 'You're not well enough to drive.' "

Undoubtedly, you'll get resistance—a lot of it—in such
a situation, again because everybody is positive they can
do it safely. Never mind the resistance, says Weslie.
"You have to say, 'I understand this happens, and it's
nothing personal. So don't feel bad. But I'm not getting
in your car and you shouldn't either.' If they go, what

can you do? It's their risk. They shouldn't take it. But if they want to, it's up to them.''

## Escape Hatch

Sometimes you can simply make a misjudgment; many of those interviewed said that, like Maggie at the top of the chapter, they got in the car with someone they thought was fine, but soon found out otherwise.

So what do you do? Your top priority must be to get out of the car. This isn't always so easy. But if you're afraid and you think the driver isn't sober, you have to try.

Sometimes the direct approach works. "I've told people to just pull over," said Allison. "That's just what you have to do sometimes."

Weslie agreed. "You have to be forceful and direct. It's no time to be polite or to beat around the bush. If the person is your friend, they'll understand." And if they don't, you need to do what you're doing anyway.

Maggie, however, is leery of too confrontational an approach. "You can't speak too derogatorily or talk down to them, because my God, you don't know what the reaction is going to be. The person has been drinking. They might get violent or angry and lose control." Maggie tries to be firm but subtle, suggesting the driver pull over. She'll say, "Are you tired?" or "Maybe we should pull over and I'll drive." Anything, she says, "to encourage them to stop the car."

There are instances, though, when nothing is working. What to do then? Said Leslie, "The one I hear about that always works is telling them you have to go to the bathroom. Either that, or that you have to throw up. Drunk as they are, they don't want you throwing up in their car." You get the driver to pull over. Once stopped, you can do your business (or fake doing it), and explain to the driver that you prefer to go on your own from here. "Or if you really need to, you can just take off," said Leslie.

The best approach of all, of course, is the preventive one; that is, being extra judicious in deciding who you drive with. But if your judgment lapses, do anything you can to get the driver to stop, for his or her sake, and yours. It may not be easy; there may be hard feelings. But your life is certainly worth some temporary hard feelings, isn't it? "Besides," said Allison, "if the person is really a friend, he'll almost always thank you later."

## Summing Up

Perhaps the most insidious aspect about drinking and driving is that it is so easy to do. You're out somewhere, you've had a few, you want to go—and you're sure you're fine. You're positive nothing will happen. You don't want to hurt yourself or anyone else. You just want to go home. So you promise yourself you'll be careful and you hit the road.

Maybe you'll get there. But maybe you won't. Just know that you're messing with a loaded weapon. And that your chances of having an accident are vastly greater than they would be normally, even if you've only had one or two.

If you can keep just one thing in mind about all this, keep what we talked about earlier: Alcohol lies. It makes you think you're fine. It makes you positive of this. It says, "No problem. Let's go. I drive very cautiously when I've had a little. I can do it. I swear I can."

It's all a lie. It's the voice of the booze, and it's a gross and vicious distortion. Because nobody drives better drunk, or high. You drive after you drink, you have a much greater chance of dying. It's that tragic, and that simple.

Hundreds of thousands of tragedies have befallen people because of this lie. Stopping and thinking about this can help prevent you from becoming a statistic, too.

"Since my accident, my brothers have gone to two parties," said Jerry. "Each time they got drunk. And each time they didn't drive. They would've if it hadn't been for what happened to me. I know it."

Jerry paused. Being the victim of a drunken-driving accident was the worst experience of his life. He had seizures and trauma and damn near lost a friend. Knowing that talking about it may help others avoid a similar fate seemed to ease the pain some.

"What my brothers did, that made me feel very good," said Jerry.

# Chapter 8

# CHANGING WHAT YOU CAN
## Coping with Someone Else's Drinking Problem

He tried everything. And anything. Peter didn't care what it took. He just knew that he really cared for Lisa and that he badly wanted to help her. Lisa definitely needed the help.

Sometimes, Peter would try talking to her. He would be very direct and honest. He would say, "You have a drinking problem and I really think you need to look at that." Other times his approach had more urgency. He would almost plead with her to face the problem: "Can't you see what this is doing to your life?"

He also would try being on his best behavior. He thought, "Well, if I'm amazingly nice to her, maybe she'll just feel better about things and not need to drink." This had the same result as everything else Peter tried: It didn't work. He'd give it his all and it would get nowhere and then he would just get frustrated. And angry.

That's when he would give Lisa the cold shoulder or hang up on her or threaten to break up. Other times he would just holler at her. Maybe that would make it sink in, make her stop, he thought.

## The Booze Spills Over

Peter learned, in a painful way, how hard it can be when you're close to someone who has a drinking problem. We're going to look at this issue in this chapter: at what can help and can't help; at what you can do to make the situation more manageable, to make yourself feel better, even if the drinker you care for is still at it.

It's very important to do this, because when you're close to someone who drinks too much, it can affect you far more than you may think. Just as the alcoholic is obsessed with drinking, we can become obsessed with stopping him. In extreme cases, especially when the drinker we're concerned about is in the immediate family, it's very easy for the drinking to become the main focus of your life. You find yourself constantly worrying about whether he's drinking, and how much; about if he'll be okay to drive home; about if his boss will find out about the drinking, or if he'll be sober when you have friends over. You can easily slip into hunting around for bottles, drawing lines on them to see how much he's had, and any number of other things. Your life can get as wrapped up around the bottle as the alcoholic's. The fact is, when you live with an alcoholic, as I did for thirteen years, you become sick, too. This is why it's called the family disease. And why it's vital to learn what you can do to stop it from totally overtaking your life.

## The Power Struggle

The first fact we need to face is that we can't control someone else's drinking. We can certainly try, as Peter did, and as I did, too. But it's futile. Pounding our heads against the wall would get us just as far.

It's hard to accept this powerlessness but very important to do so. The longer we go on thinking we can— indeed, should—be able to do something about the problem, the more we leave ourselves open to hurt, guilt (for not being successful), and tons of frustration. I carried them all for a long time, until I started going to Alateen and Al-Anon (support groups for people whose lives are being affected by someone else's drinking), and until I gradually came to grips with what I was up against. It was no fun.

## Mission Impossible

More than anything else, I wanted to get my mother to stop drinking. It was ruining my life, her life, the whole family's life. I, too, pleaded and begged. I tried being extra nice and devoted. If she wanted company, I stayed home. If she felt like going somewhere, I'd go with her. Like Peter, I figured if I could help make her more contented, the less she would need booze.

There were frequent promises to stop. Sometimes she actually *would* stop. But always, it would start back up again.

No matter how well-conceived and well-intentioned they may be, our efforts to stop or limit someone else's drinking will lead us nowhere. The reason is that people who can't control their drinking are alcoholics. They have the disease of alcoholism. They are powerless over their drinking, because it is a physiological compulsion, and a psychological one as well. They're terrified to live without it, while the reality is they can't live with it.

We can try loving the disease out of them or shaming it out of them. We can ignore them, scream at them, or coddle them. We can pour out bottles—I've emptied more than a few—or dilute the supply with water. We can have heart-to-heart talks with them.

None of these sorts of things work, any more than Darrin's mother bribing him with a motorcycle worked. That's because we're up against a disease, and this is not how diseases are treated.

## A Healthy Detachment

Weslie was worried about her friend, Amy. Very worried. "She was getting ripped every night," said Weslie. "We'd have a little get-together and everyone would drink a little, and she would wind up on the floor. It was like the wine cooler bottle was melted to her hand. It got so everyone would get mad."

Weslie tried approaching Amy. "I'd say, 'Why do you drink so much?' And she would say because it made her feel good and because she wanted to escape. I'd say, 'Why don't you give me the bottle? It's not good to drink that way.' "

Weslie was angry at Amy for her drinking, and she got even angrier when Amy started blaming others—Weslie included—saying they were the ones who always got her the wine coolers. "I haven't talked to her since," said Weslie.

Weslie's reaction is very understandable, and practically universal. You care for someone, you want them to stop drinking. When they don't, you feel hurt and let down. You get angry. You blame them, maybe lash out at them. You think they're just being stubborn or acting like jerks.

This is where remembering that this is a disease comes in. We do ourselves a big favor when we learn not to take the drinking personally, when we accept that the drinker has this terrible compulsion, and they're drinking not because they have no willpower or because they deliberately want to hurt us but because they simply cannot control it.

Stepping back from the drinking in this way is called detachment. It's very hard to do, precisely because it is so easy to take the drinking personally. We see the alcoholic drinking, we know it's doing big damage to them, and we just want to scream, "Would you just can it already? What are you doing to yourself?" It sure seems like it's a question of willpower; it seems like they should be able to just stop. But it's not that easy. Not by a long shot.

## Hold the Blame

Like Weslie, Karen is very angry. Her mother is an alcoholic. "She says she drinks because she has problems," said Karen. "I say, 'Why don't you talk to somebody? Why don't you talk to us?' She says, 'No, nobody can help me.' So she drinks. She won't admit she has a problem. She denies it. She blames all of us. She even blames the pets. We don't listen, we don't love her, we don't care."

Karen said, "My mother wants everybody to feel sorry for her. She doesn't care about us." You can hear Karen's hurt.

Allison has an alcoholic brother. She speaks of him and you see her pain very clearly, too. Her voice quivers, then turns sharp and harsh. "I hate him for what he's done," she said. "I wouldn't care if I never saw him again. All he's done is cause the family pain. He breaks into the house, he steals, lies. He's a bum. He has made my mother a wreck. All he cares about is his next drink."

It's very easy to want to blame the alcoholic for his drinking. I felt, deep down, that if my mother really wanted to, she would stop getting wasted every night. I just kept thinking, "If she loved me she would stop."

But the loving and the stopping have nothing to do with one another. As understandable as it is, blaming the alcoholic for drinking does no good at all. In fact, it can do a lot of harm. Because no matter how he acts overtly— even if he's hostile or defiant or seeming without remorse—the problem drinker is crammed full of guilt. This is a deeply buried feeling, but it's there. I've lived with a few problem drinkers, and interviewed many more. Over and over, I've heard them say, "Deep down, I hated myself for the drinking. I felt worthless. I hated what I was doing to myself and my family and friends. But I was terrified. I couldn't stop." Our blaming, on top of the guilt that's already there and growing by the drink, only makes the alcoholic's burden heavier. And because of the added burden, it only makes them want to drink more. That, after all, is the only way they have of coping with things.

Allison's brother and Karen's mother, like all alcoholics—are sick people. Their sickness has made their lives totally unmanageable. Lying, stealing, deceiving— this is common behavior for alcoholics, because the sickness overpowers everything else in their life. As Allison said, "All the alcoholic cares about is where his next drink is coming from." That's just about right.

## Barrooms and Bullets

One alcoholic related a story of one of his hundreds of late-night stints in a bar. The owner wanted to close and head home. This fellow, however, wasn't ready to leave. The owner kept badgering him. Sam, the drinker, stayed put.

Finally, the bar owner came over and stuck a gun in Sam's gut. He said, "It's time for you to go home." Sam, who is about six five and 240 pounds, stood up. He grabbed the gun and turned it away and said right in the face of the owner, "We're going to have another round and it's on me."

Sam got his final round. It wasn't until a few days later—"when I sobered up," he said—that he realized what he had done. "I didn't think anything of it at the time," he said. "But all of a sudden it hit me, and I started shaking thinking about it." Drinking was the top thing—the only thing—on Sam's agenda. Even a gun to the belly wasn't going to change it.

This is how insane the disease can get. And it is this very insanity that, for our own sanity, we need to detach from. Instead of blaming or keeping track of all the awful things the alcoholic does, it's much more constructive to just accept that the alcoholic has a very wicked disease. We can still love the alcoholic, even as we learn to hate his disease. We can do this by learning about the affliction, and by working at not getting hurt. So when the drinker lies to us, or promises to do us a favor and goes and gets drunk instead, or any number of other things, we can say, "This person is sick. The drinking is ruling his life. He is not doing this to hurt me."

# Weathering the Onslaught

Detaching is never harder than when the problem drinker is passing blame or hostility in our direction. Weslie told of her friend Amy blaming her friends for getting it for her. Karen related how her mother blamed Karen and everyone else in the family for mistreating her.

Ellen's father is an alcoholic. "He's a really nice guy when he's sober," she said. "But when he's drunk, he's a monster. He blames my brother and me for everything. He says things like, 'You were my two biggest mistakes. I wish you'd never been born.' What are you supposed to do?" Ellen paused. She said, "That really hurts me."

Karen heard Ellen relate this, and added, "Alcoholics like to put people down. My mother puts us down all the time, especially my sister. She'll say things like, 'I'm not going to leave you anything in the will,' just deliberate things to hurt you."

Many alcoholics *do* like to put others down, particularly those close to them. They also like to do a lot of blaming for their plight.

It's important to recognize that this behavior springs from the misery the alcoholic feels about what is happening. Low self-esteem is a big, ugly part of this disease. The problem drinker loathes what he's doing to himself and those who are closest to him. The pain gets to be too much, and one of the unfortunate ways of dealing with it is to spread the misery around.

Audrey was talking about her life when her mother was drinking heavily, all day, every day. Audrey had just had the most traumatic experience in her life—an abortion. She had never felt more fragile. She was undergoing therapy and her guilt was heavy and life at home was hell. Audrey needed support. She needed a lot of it. What she got, when her mother was drunk, was a stream of vicious barbs about murdering the child. The cliche is true: Misery loves company. The disease makes the alcoholic want to drag everybody down with him.

Hearing such things obviously isn't pleasant. Indeed, it can be brutal. But it helps greatly to remember that this is really the disease doing the talking. Again, the key is to detach, to separate our real friend or parent from the diseased individual. In the vast majority of cases, the awful things we hear are not meant, even remotely. It's just the sickness doing its sinister work.

Practicing detachment gives protection. It fortifies us with a kind of emotional armor. So the next time you hear some venomous, drunken rambling, you can tell yourself, "This is the disease talking. I need to pull back from this. I don't have to get upset by this." By focusing on our own reactions, rather than the nasty words, we can do a whole lot for our peace of mind.

## Letting Go of Blame

This process is important in another regard as well, in that it helps us not dwell on the guilt we're getting bombarded with. It's very easy, when you hear yourself getting blamed all the time, to begin to believe it; to think, "Maybe he is drinking because I'm a rotten kid." Or, "Maybe it is my fault because I wanted to break up with him." You need to remember—and never forget: *Someone else's drinking is not your fault.* We've all got plenty of shortcomings. But whatever yours may be, they cannot make someone else an alcoholic. They cannot drive someone else into a compulsion. The drinker may want us to think this is true, but it's not. And if we don't keep reminding ourselves of that, it's frightfully easy to feel pretty awful inside.

## Dealing with Denial

Alcoholics are great at finding scapegoats for their drinking. They will blame anyone and anything. A girlfriend or boyfriend problem, an unfaithful spouse, a kid getting in trouble, difficulties at school or work, money worries—you name it, the alcoholic can use it to blame his drinking problem on.

Remember, alcoholics are terrified to think their drinking is out of control. It is their ultimate fear, and the blaming is an effective way to get around it, to reinforce the drinker's diseased inner voice, which is saying, even as he's getting himself into major messes, "You don't have a problem. You can control your drinking. Everybody's making a big deal out of nothing." The voice also says, "Go ahead. Have a drink. You'll feel better."

The rationalizations for drinking are almost endless. Possibly you've heard one of these:

- "If everybody would stop hassling me about it, everything would be fine."
- "I'm just going through a tough time right now."
- "If you had my problems you would drink, too."
- "Drinking isn't my problem; you're my problem."

Or the drinker may come up with more specific reasons: "I really blew that midterm," or "I just found out Jessica's been two-timing me." The drinker will latch onto anything at all.

Denial can be one of the hardest things to deal with. Of her friend Amy, Weslie said, "It made me so mad. How could she not see what was happening?" Peter, too, would go crazy sometimes, because Lisa refused to admit her problem. She would make excuses or just blow the whole issue off. Peter couldn't believe it. It was as though she were living in another world. And in a sense, that's exactly right; that is how much the denial can distort the drinker's perceptions. For a good eight years, one alcoholic I know insisted he had other problems—with his wife, with his kids—but not one with alcohol. He clung to this, even in the face of a shattered marriage, blackouts, a stay in a mental institution, suicide attempts, and more. There's no overestimating how powerful denial can be.

With denial, too, it's vital for us to keep in mind it's the work of the disease. The drinker is not just lying to us for the heck of it, or refusing to face things so everyone else will go insane from frustration. It's simply a product of that voice: "Hey, you don't have a problem."

As easy as it is to get hurt and angry about this, we can protect ourselves. We can work at accepting the denial as part of the illness, at not allowing ourselves to get consumed by these feelings. It's hard, sure, but rather than have our lives beaten down because a friend won't face this problem, we can focus on understanding things on a deeper level. We can make ourselves much less frustrated over it. We can do it by accepting that only when things get bad enough and painful enough will the denial be pierced, and will the alcoholic face the harsh reality of things.

## Hitting Bottom

Lisa, Peter's friend, has not had anything to drink in nearly six months. All his efforts to get her to stop, as we've seen, did nothing. What it took was for Lisa to see the extent of the problem for herself.

"I denied it for a long time," Lisa said. "I would say, 'I don't have a problem. I just like to drink. So what's wrong with that?' My boyfriend would talk to me, and another friend would, too. I said, 'No, no, no. I just like feeling good.'

"It took a long time," Lisa went on, "but eventually it sank in." She started drinking more often, just about every day after school. She would drink at home, alone. She made vows to stop, just to prove she could do it. The vows would always get broken. "I would say I would only have one beer, and then I would have another and another. I would start and I just couldn't stop."

Lisa's denial started crumbling. What brought it down altogether was her brother. She saw him drunk one day. He was really drunk. He was wild. Lisa was sober at the time. "I just watched him, and it made me really scared." The fear hit home. Suddenly, she could see not only what alcohol was doing to someone she loved, but also what it was doing to her. Lisa was ready to get help, to get sober. She started speaking to a counselor. She talked to friends about her drinking. She opened up with her brother, sharing her realization about her own problem, and also her concern about his. Lisa admitted that drinking was causing problems in her life. And this is the first giant step toward getting sober.

It's very difficult to stand by and watch someone we care for hit bottom. Often this may involve a bad fight or an accident or a hospitalization, as was the case with Darrin. But this is frequently what is necessary for the drinker to seek help. We can't talk them into getting sober, or force them to see the reality of things. They need to see it for themselves; only then will they truly be motivated to get help.

Peter and Lisa's case is the classic example. He did

everything he could think of to get her sober. But nothing changed until she hit her bottom and accepted that things really did need changing.

## What We Can Do

We've talked a lot in this chapter about things we shouldn't, or can't, do in relating to a problem drinker. We've looked at not trying to control the drinking and not blaming the drinker and not taking the lies and insults and blaming to heart. But is there any active step we can take to help the drinker see his problem?

For one thing, we can talk to the person. We can be candid and direct about it, as long as we don't preach or become judgmental. It won't get us anywhere to say, "Everybody thinks you're turning into the town drunk," or, "You're really disappointing me."

But it may do some good to say something straight and simple, such as, "I'm concerned about your drinking," or "I've been worried about you lately." A plain, direct statement from a good friend may well give the drinker something to think about.

This is not an easy thing to do. As Rita said, "How do you say something like that? I think that would be about the hardest thing to talk to someone about." Nor are there guarantees it'll do any good. He may ignore you, or accuse you of overreacting or tell you to mind your own business. But approaching him in this way couldn't hurt, and you never know: It could help. At the very least, you're giving him something to mull over. And even if he keeps on drinking for the time being, there's no telling when your honesty may combine with other warning signals and help the drinker begin to see the damage that's being done.

If you do choose to approach the person, remember never to try it when he's been drinking. That's the worst time. You never know what his response will be while he's under the influence. You don't even know how much he'll remember of your talk. Do it when he's straight. There's still no certainty about his reaction, but at least you'll know you're dealing with an unpolluted mind.

## Call Off the Rescue Squad

Another thing we can do that will help the problem drinker is learning not to rescue him from his alcohol-made messes.

Say, for instance, you have a friend whose drinking you're worried about. Suppose her name is Hillary, and that lately at parties, she's gotten quite belligerent after she's on her way, and she's alienating more and more of her friends. You're very loyal to Hillary. You hate to see her getting herself in trouble. So you dutifully go around to all the offended parties and do your best to patch things up and let everybody know that Hillary's just going through a tough time and that she really doesn't mean to be acting this way.

In this scenario, your intentions are very noble. But your results could well be far from noble. They might only make Hillary's drinking problem worse. Because by undoing some of the damage her drinking is causing, you are, in effect, making it easier for her to continue denying the problem.

## Helping by Not Helping

We know problem drinkers will deny things as long as they can. By rescuing them, or enabling them, as it is often called (in the sense of *enabling* them to continue drinking), all we're doing is insulating them from the consequences of their alcohol abuse. As long as they're protected, how will they ever hit bottom?

Not enabling is a tough challenge. It may have been the single toughest thing about the disease for me. It meant that if my mother passed out on the floor, I would leave her there to sleep. It meant refusing to call in sick for her if she couldn't work, and not preparing meals for her if she hadn't been sober enough to eat food in a day and a half. When you really care for someone, not doing these things seems almost impossible at first. It seems cruel and selfish and heartless. But it's in the best interests of the problem drinker, and that's the thing we need to continually tell ourselves. We are not being heartless at all. In the big picture, in fact, we're doing the kindest thing we can. We're letting the alcoholic clean up his own messes, whatever they may be. And maybe, as a result of one of these messes, he will see that drinking is ruining his life. And then, maybe, he'll get help.

This works, believe me. My mother accepted that she had this terrible problem only after all of us enablers stopped enabling. Our message to her was, "Mom, we love you, but we're not going to rescue you from your drinking." We didn't stop being nice to her, or being as kind and supportive family members as we could; we just stopped the rescuing.

She didn't like it, not one bit, at first. Alcoholics usually don't, particularly when they're used to getting enabled. But it helped her in a way that all the enabling kindnesses in the world could not have.

So let's go back to your friend, Hillary. Suppose, after she's spent most of the weekend—and all of her money— boozing it up, she comes up to you and asks if you can advance her some money. You say, "I'm sorry, I can't help you out right now." No lecture is necessary ("You blew your money on liquor, that's why"), or appropriate. All you need to do is say no. If she presses, you can tell her exactly what your feeling is: that you're concerned about her drinking and you don't want to fuel it in any way.

Or maybe Hillary has been partying so much she has fallen behind in her studies. Suddenly there's a term paper due and she's barely opened a book. She needs your help. She asks for your notes, wants you to help her catch up and get her started on the paper. Again, you respectfully decline.

Is this tough to put into action? You bet. But it's a darn good cause. Causes don't come much better than helping somebody you care for escape the ravages of alcoholism.

## A Final Thought

There's one more thing you can do for yourself if you're troubled by someone else's drinking. And that is to understand that there's nothing whatsoever for you to be embarrassed or ashamed about.

Such feelings can be very prevalent and powerful, particularly if the drinker is one of your parents. You may be ashamed to bring friends over to the house. You may look at other mothers or fathers and wish yours could be like that. You may live in steady fear of neighbors finding out about what goes on inside your home. I remember once my mother insisted on going to a meet-the-teachers session at my school, even though she had been drinking. I thought of her meeting my teachers in such a state, and I wanted to head for the hills.

But as I came to accept the disease concept, I also began to accept that sickness is nothing to be ashamed about. It's a terrible disease, but it's also a very common one. The fact that my parent had this addiction does not make me less of a person, or any less worthy of having a good life. If my teachers held it against me, well, I would just have to deal with that. All it would really show, in any case, is that they're pretty ignorant.

Whether you have a family member or friend whose drinking concerns you, keep in mind that it is no reflection on you. There is nothing about it that has anything to do with you. You would be very saddened, of course, if somebody close to you developed cancer or some other disease. But you wouldn't feel shame about it, and wouldn't think it showed that you were a bad person. You shouldn't feel that about the disease of alcoholism, either.

It's also worth remembering that, if you are affected by someone's drinking, you are a long way from being alone. You may feel alone, and feel that nobody could know what it's like or how much it hurts or how crazy it can make life. But the fact is that millions of us know all about it. One study revealed that one out of three Americans reported being affected by someone else's drinking.

So if you are living with this problem, work at what we've talked about. Work at detaching from the disease, and keep at it, because it isn't easy. And remember: There's a huge work force, millions of us, who are out there with you.

# EPILOGUE

The names are pretty familiar to you by now. They are Jerry and Allison and Maggie and Evan, and dozens of others. They're the voices you've just heard from—the teenagers who made this book by sharing their thoughts on drinking, on any and all aspects of it.

They've talked about when they started drinking, and why. Some of them talked about the appeal of drinking, some others about why they find no appeal in it at all. They looked at using alcohol to escape and at feeling pressure to drink, and how they deal with their parents when it comes to drinking. They talked about getting drunk and getting hung over and how alcohol affected them; three of them talked about how they started drinking and couldn't stop and had to come face to face with the frightening reality of their alcoholism.

We've looked at how alcohol works over the body and

the mind; at what it does when it's inside you, and how it finally leaves. We've heard from a lot of people about how hard it is when someone you care for has a drinking problem. And we've heard from just about everybody on maybe the most critical matter of all: drinking and driving.

Some of the voices belong to young people whose watchword is caution. These are people who respect and/or fear alcohol, and don't want to get mixed up in it at all. Others you've heard from enjoy drinking in moderation, and still others lean more toward the wild; they like to party and show no hesitation about it. A few don't just lean that way—they're fully camped there.

## Heeding the Voices

You've heard thoughts and feelings and attitudes of virtually every flavor, from all kinds of people. That was the aim going in, not just for variety's sake, but to pack in as much "straight talk" as possible. It made sense that the more voices that were put in the more you would have to take out. And that, after all, is why this book was written: To give you some things—some important things—to hold on to, things to filter through your mind *before* you put your lips to a bottle.

The hope is that, in hearing these voices and considering what they had to say, you learned some things about alcohol, and gained some facts and insights you didn't have before. The hope also is that what you learned has given you a sense of why your decisions about alcohol—whether to drink, when to drink, how to drink—are among the most important choices you have to make. More than anything else, the point of gathering all these voices was to help you understand that thinking hard about all this is one of the smartest things you can do.

In the Introduction, I told of how little forethought I gave my own alcohol use, and how dumb this was. The book will have been a success if you don't follow my lead; if you consider what the voices have said, and if you recognize this is a serious matter with potentially serious consequences; if you realize that the firm belief that an alcohol problem could never happen to you is no protection whatsoever. You think that, I think that, we all do. And we're all wrong. Because alcoholism could happen to any one of us. We don't know. Which is exactly why this whole issue *is* so serious.

The parting thought, then, is a very simple one: Think about it. Think hard about it. Just the way Maggie thinks about it:

"I know a lot of people who don't think about drinking much. Those are the people who are at every party, getting drunk. And I think those are the ones that don't care about themselves enough.

"That's what a lot of it is," said Maggie. "I care about myself. I want to think about it. I think if you do care about yourself, it's the only way to go."

# APPENDIX
## Getting Help

Have you ever thought you might have a drinking problem?

It's a simple, direct question. It can be hard to answer.

Below is a test that aims to help. It has been devised by the National Council on Alcoholism, and its purpose is to help identify if a problem exists. Give it a shot. Be as honest as you can be. Fudging answers isn't going to get you anywhere, except to prolong the trouble alcohol may be causing you and to make the situation harder to deal with at some future point.

Yes  No

☐   ☐   1. Do you occasionally drink heavily after a disappointment, a quarrel, or when the boss gives you a hard time?

☐ ☐ 2. When you have trouble or feel under pressure, do you always drink more heavily than usual?

☐ ☐ 3. Have you noticed that you are able to handle more liquor than you did when you were first drinking?

☐ ☐ 4. Did you ever wake up on the "morning after" and discover that you could not remember part of the evening before, even though your friends tell you that you did not "pass out"?

☐ ☐ 5. When drinking with other people, do you try to have a few extra drinks when others will not know it?

☐ ☐ 6. Are there certain occasions when you feel uncomfortable if alcohol is not available?

☐ ☐ 7. Have you recently noticed that when you begin drinking you are in more of a hurry to get the first drink than you used to be?

☐ ☐ 8. Do you sometimes feel a little guilty about your drinking?

☐ ☐ 9. Are you secretly irritated when your family or friends discuss your drinking?

☐ ☐ 10. Have you recently noticed an increase in the frequency of your memory "blackouts"?

☐ ☐ 11. Do you often find that you wish to continue drinking after your friends say they have had enough?

☐ ☐ 12. Do you usually have a reason for the occasions when you drink heavily?

☐ ☐ 13. When you are sober, do you often regret things you have done or said while drinking?

☐ ☐ 14. Have you tried switching brands or following different plans for controlling your drinking?

☐ ☐ 15. Have you often failed to keep the promises you have made to yourself about controlling or cutting down on your drinking?

☐  ☐   16. Have you ever tried to control your drinking by making a change in jobs, or moving to a new location?

☐  ☐   17. Do you try to avoid family or close friends while you are drinking?

☐  ☐   18. Are you having an increasing number of financial and work problems?

☐  ☐   19. Do more people seem to be treating you unfairly without good reason?

☐  ☐   20. Do you eat very little or irregularly when you are drinking?

☐  ☐   21. Do you sometimes have the "shakes" in the morning and find that it helps to have a little drink?

☐  ☐   22. Have you recently noticed that you cannot drink as much as you once did?

☐  ☐   23. Do you sometimes stay drunk for several days at a time?

☐  ☐   24. Do you sometimes feel very depressed and wonder whether life is worth living?

☐  ☐   25. Sometimes after periods of drinking, do you see or hear things that aren't there?

☐  ☐   26. Do you get terribly frightened after you have been drinking heavily?

Any "yes" answer indicates a probable symptom of alcoholism.

"Yes" answers to several of the questions indicate the following stages of alcoholism:

Questions 1–8—Early stage.
Questions 9–21—Middle stage.
Questions 22–26—The beginning of final stage.

National Council on Alcoholism. Reprinted with permission.

# If You're Concerned About Your Drinking

Where should you turn if you do have a drinking problem? The first—and in my view, the best—choice is Alcoholics Anonymous. As noted in the text, A.A. is a support group for alcoholics that meets in hundreds of thousands of communities around the world. There is almost certainly an A.A. group near you. Typically, meetings are held in a local church or community building. If you live in or near or good-sized town or city, chances are there are several meetings every day. They cost nothing and are made up solely of alcoholics who are "working the A.A. program," as they say, helping one another get sober and stay sober. As the name suggests, anonymity is totally guarded at these meetings.

If you have a problem—even if you're not sure—try an A.A. meeting. Try going to several of them, in fact. You will be welcomed warmly (most meetings have newcomers all the time), and you will be joining a group that has helped more people recover from alcoholism than all other treatment programs combined. A.A. has a saying, "You're in the right place," and indeed, if you have a drinking problem, you are. The organization was founded by alcoholics and exists solely to help alcoholics. It is a brotherhood (and sisterhood) of people helping one another achieve recovery, one day at a time.

If you can't get to a meeting, or if you feel awkward about going, the next best step is to find someone to talk to. If you look in the white pages under Alcoholics Anonymous (or call information), you can probably get a number to call so you can talk to an A.A. member about your problem before even setting foot in a meeting. Looking under the heading "Alcoholism" might put you in touch with other helping organizations in your area. You also might try talking to your parents, the school social worker, a clergyman, or a teacher you feel you can trust. Your parents would usually be the first choice, but if your relationship with them makes you uncomfortable talking with them about your drinking right now, find someone else. But find someone. It's very important to reach out to an adult. You'll feel better having shared the problem, and you also will have recruited an ally to help you help yourself—someone who might be able to drive you to a meeting, or just listen to you, or make other suggestions about where to go for support and help in your community.

Talking to someone about your drinking problem can be very hard at the beginning. But trust that you are doing the right thing. It's the first big step toward getting better.

## Al-Anon and More: Other Helping Hands

What if you're being affected by someone else's drinking—a parent, another family member, a friend? A.A.'s companion organization, Al-Anon, is the best route to go here, too. Alateen is the teenage component of Al-Anon, which, as we've discussed, is a wonderful support group whose whole reason for being, just as A.A.'s is to help the drinker, is to help those of us who live with (or are close to) a problem drinker.

Alateen meetings are not gripe or gossip sessions; they are not gatherings where young people get together and talk about how awful their drinking parents and friends are. They are simply meetings at which people share their experiences and hopes, and nurture one another as they follow the Al-Anon program's outlook to let go of obsessions about the drinker and focus, instead, on doing things for yourself.

There is nothing to feel guilty about in going to Alateen; you're not tattling on the alcoholic. You are there to help yourself deal with a family disease. Here, too, anonymity is the foundation of the program. You go to these meetings to get help. And from my experiences, you can get more help at Al-Anon than anywhere.

To locate a group in or near your community, look under Al-Anon in the white pages, or under Alcoholism in the yellow pages. If that doesn't work, look under Alcoholics Anonymous in the white pages or call information; the A.A. people should be happy to let you know when and where Al-Anon/Alateen meets in the area.

Here again, if getting to a meeting is a problem, or if you feel uncomfortable about it, find an adult you trust, and talk to him or her. Share your concerns and your feelings. Talk about what you're going through. Try to get hold of reading material; the Al-Anon listing is one place to turn, if a counselor or another trusted adult cannot help you. And again, do your best to get to a few Alateen meetings. You're bound to feel a little awkward at first; I certainly did. But if you give it a chance, you come to see that you're surrounded by people who are coping with the same hurt and anger and crises that you are. Coping right along with them is about the greatest comfort you can find.

A.A. and Al-Anon both have a wide variety of very helpful reading material, ranging from thin pamphlets to fat books. For more information, write or call:

Alcoholics Anonymous
General Service Office
P.O. Box 459

Grand Central Station
New York, NY 10163
(212) 686-1100

Al-Anon Family Group Headquarters
P.O. Box 182
Madison Square Station
New York, NY 10159
(212) 302-7240

Hazleden, the alcohol and drug rehabilitation center in Center City, Minnesota, also publishes much helpful information. For details, call (800) 328-9000 (outside Minnesota), or (800) 257-0070 (within Minnesota).

Plume _____ (0452)

# FEELING GOOD

☐ **GOOD HANDS: MASSAGE TECHNIQUES FOR TOTAL HEALTH by Robert Bahr.**
This comprehensive introduction to the art and science of massage teaches classical massage, finger pressure massage, deep friction massage and connective tissue massage. With detailed drawings and step-by-step instructions. Relieve tired muscles, stop painful spasms and prevent injuries with Bahr's professional methods.
(256089—$8.95)

☐ **DARE TO CHANGE: How to Program Yourself for Success, by Joe Alexander.**
Most people never come close to fulfilling their potential for achievement and happiness. They are held back not by outside forces—but by the "inner saboteurs" that have been programmed into them since childhood and that cripple their ability to see, think, and act. This innovative guide to discovery and growth will prove that you have the power to direct your own life—and make your future better than your past.
(255309—$7.95)

☐ **FAMILY COMMUNICATION (Revised Edition), by Sven Wahlroós, Ph.D.** An innovative guide to successful family living, it will teach you and your family how to achieve emotional health, warmer feelings, and closer, more loving relationships.
(254604—$8.95)

☐ **THE COMPLETE GUIDE TO WOMEN'S HEALTH by Bruce D. Shephard, M.D. and Carroll A. Shephard, R.N., Ph.D.** The most comprehensive, up-to-date resource available for making vital health decisions ... advice on diet fitness; 135 common symptoms from A to Z, explained and referenced ... "Excellent, informative ... beautifully organized"—Jane Brody, *The New York Times.*          (256739—$11.95)

_____

Prices slightly higher in Canada.
_____

Buy them at your local bookstore or use this convenient
coupon for ordering.

**NEW AMERICAN LIBRARY**
**P.O. Box 999, Bergenfield, New Jersey 07621**

Please send me the PLUME BOOKS I have checked above. I am enclosing
$_____ (please add $1.50 to this order to cover postage and handling). Send check or money order—no cash or C.O.D.'s. Prices and numbers are subject to change without notice.

Name_____

Address_____

City_____ State_____ Zip Code_____

Allow 4-6 weeks for delivery.
This offer is subject to withdrawal without notice.